THE MAUDSLEY

PRESCRIBING GUIDELINES

The Maudsley

The South London and Maudsley NHS Trust

2001
PRESCRIBING
GUIDELINES

6th Edition

<table>
<tr><td>David Taylor</td><td>Denise McConnell</td></tr>
<tr><td>Harry McConnell</td><td>Robert Kerwin</td></tr>
</table>

MARTIN DUNITZ

© Taylor, McConnell, McConnell, Kerwin 2001

First published in the United Kingdom in 1999 by

Martin Dunitz Ltd
The Livery House
7–9 Pratt Street
London NW1 0AE

Tel: +44 (0) 20-7482-2202
Fax: +44 (0) 20-7267-0159
E-mail: info.dunitz@tandf.co.uk
Website: http://www.dunitz.co.uk

Fifth edition 1999
Sixth edition 2001

Reprinted 2001

A CIP record for this book is available from the British Library.

ISBN 1–85317–963–9

Distributed in the United States by:
Blackwell Science Inc.
Commerce Place, 350 Main Street
Malden, MA 02148, USA
Tel: +1–800–215–1000

Distributed in Canada by:
Login Brothers Book Company
324 Salteaux Crescent
Winnipeg, Manitoba, R3J 3T2
Canada
Tel: +1–204–224–4068

Distributed in Brazil by:
Ernesto Reichmann Distribuidora de Livros, Ltda
Rua Coronel Marques 335, Tatuape 03440–000
Sao Paulo,
Brazil

Printed and bound in Italy by Printer Trento

Authors and editors

David Taylor, Senior Editor and Lead Author
Chief Pharmacist, South London and Maudsley NHS Trust
Honorary Senior Lecturer, Institute of Psychiatry

Harry McConnell, Author
Psychiatrist and neurologist
Clinical Editor
BMJ Publishing Group

Denise Duncan-McConnell, Author
Principal Clinical Pharmacist, South London and Maudsley NHS Trust

Robert Kerwin, Founding Editor
Professor of Clinical Neuropharmacology, Institute of Psychiatry
Consultant Psychiatrist, South London and Maudsley NHS Trust

Disclaimer

The opinions expressed are those of the individual authors in consultation with various international experts and with the South London and Maudsley NHS Trust's Drug and Therapeutics Committee. Every care has been taken to assure that these Guidelines are up-to-date and accurate. However, it must be considered that this document is but the end product of reasoned influences from several clinicians. We do not claim that every piece of advice provided is "correct", only that we have taken care to ensure that advice is based on firm evidence and clinical experience. We hope to have included all information available to us in August 2000, but this will inevitably become outdated as time goes by. Readers should bear this in mind and should always consult the latest manufacturers' information and the British National Formulary or the equivalent text for their country of practice.

It is also important to recognise that Clinical Practice differs from one country to another and that availability and licensing of drugs discussed in these Guidelines also vary with geographical location. Please note that many of the drugs listed in the tables are done so alphabetically and not necessarily in order of preference. Generic drugs may require special care and attention in relation to dosage and use. Special attention should always be paid to contraindications and side effects. Many of the drugs discussed are not yet available in some countries and many of the uses may be "off licence" in the UK as well as overseas. Similarly, recommended doses vary greatly from country to country. Clinicians are strongly advised to check their local laws and local hospital or national clinical guidelines before using any information in a clinical situation. The clinical care of any individual patient remains at all times that of the treating psychiatrist or other clinician. Additional terms and conditions may apply and may be notified. All regulatory bodies will be those of the United Kingdom and the law of England will apply in all matters relating to the Maudsley Prescribing Guidelines. No liability is accepted for any injury, loss or damage howsoever caused.

Contents

V Treatment of Special Patient Populations

Preface

Prescribing medicines is an increasingly complex and demanding process. This is especially true in psychiatry where the artistry and empiricism of former times is quickly being replaced by evidence-based and outcomes-led practice.

The Maudsley Prescribing Guidelines were first published in 1994, largely in recognition of the developing difficulties in choosing the right drug for the right patient. The *Guidelines* grew in size and scope through the 2nd, 3rd and 4th editions, but remained essentially a text used by the former Bethlem and Maudsley NHS Trust and by a few clinicians in other centres. The 5th edition of *The Guidelines*, published in 1999 for the first time by Martin Dunitz Ltd, gained nationwide usage, with more than 20,000 copies sold.

This 6th edition of *The Maudsley Prescribing Guidelines* has been fully updated and expanded to include data published between January 1999 and August 2000. The guidance provided is now supported by specific references, and potentially contentious recommendations are now accompanied by referenced discussion. Of course, published data do not provide answers to all prescribing dilemmas and so, where data are lacking, we have provided recommendations based on clinical experience, wide consultation and expert opinion. Both evidence-based and opinion-based recommendations are now clearly delineated in the text.

The Maudsley Prescribing Guidelines are primarily intended to be of use to prescribers and pharmacists working in secondary care. However, in this 6th edition, we have made special efforts to ensure the text is also of benefit to general practitioners and community pharmacists. We hope also that nursing staff, psychologists and occupational therapists will find the text helpful.

David Taylor
September 2000

Acknowledgements

The Maudsley Prescribing Guidelines is a product of the authors' knowledge and expertise and the helpful contributions of a large number of specialists and experts. The input from these experts not only allows a greater range of subjects to be covered but also provides crucial, if informal, peer review of many sections. We are, therefore, deeply indebted to the following contributors to *The Guidelines*.

Kathryn Abel
Sigurd Ackerman
David Baldwin
Ken Barrett
Jenny Bearn
Marika Bogyi
Stuart Checkley
Ed Coffey
Janet Darlington
Paul Farmer
Mike Farrell
Simon Fleminger
Eric Fombonne
Jat Harchowal
Isabel Heyman
Gary Hogman
Mike Isaac
Sarah Jarvis
Malcolm Lader
Simon Lovestone
Ibrahim al-Khodair

Channi Kumar
Jane Marshall
Pat McElhatton
Shameem Mir
Hilary Nissenbaum
Carol Paton
Rod Pipe
Lucy Reeves
Sarah Romans
Paramala Santosh
Kapil Sayal
Marisa Silverman
Trevor Silverstone
Peter Snyder
Eric Taylor
Mary Teasdale
Janet Treasure
Kate Trotter
David Veale
Fiona Woods
Eromona Whiskey

Special thanks also to Mrs Eileen Percival and Miss Jo Ashton

I
Principles of
Psychotropic Prescribing

General principles

+ The decision to use drug therapy must take into account the potential risks and benefits of treatment to the patient. These should be discussed with the patient and/or their carer along with treatment options. (See CAAT system in Appendix 2.)
+ A full evaluation of the patient's symptoms should be undertaken by the clinician before prescribing, including mental status and physical examination and laboratory tests. It is important to clarify the diagnosis since many illnesses may present as depression, psychosis or anxiety.
+ Use of drug combinations (polypharmacy) should be avoided whenever possible. When combination therapy is necessary, attention should be given to both pharmacodynamic and pharmacokinetic interactions and drug choices made accordingly.
+ In general, the lowest effective dose of a drug should be used.
+ Titration of most psychotropic agents should be done gradually and weaning of them should also be done slowly in chronic and subacute conditions. In acute situations, choice of drug will depend in part on how rapidly it may be titrated for a given clinical situation. The rate of titration and of weaning will vary depending on the class of drug and how long a patient has been taking the drug. One should be aware of those psychotropics which may cause a discontinuation syndrome or which may cause rebound symptoms or withdrawal phenomena.
+ In switching from one psychotropic to another the clinician must take into account the half-life of the drug being discontinued, the potential for discontinuation symptoms and any potential interactions (pharmacokinetic and pharmacodynamic) with the new agent.
+ In discontinuing psychotropics in patients one must consider the length of time a patient has been on the drug as well as the issues of physical and psychological withdrawal. For some drugs (e.g. antiepileptic drugs, benzodiazepines) it may be appropriate to withdraw agents over many months. Others may be discontinued abruptly or withdrawn over days / weeks.

Use of laboratory monitoring

The history, mental status examination and physical examination form the cornerstone of psychiatric diagnosis and are key to monitoring of prescribing and following a patient's progress. It is often necessary, however, to use a variety of laboratory tests, EEG and neuroimaging to assist in the diagnosis and treatment of psychiatric illness. The following table outlines some of the more helpful blood tests and their relevance to psychiatric practice.

Laboratory tests and their relevance in psychiatry

(modified from McConnell 1998)

Test	Comments
WBC count and differential	Important for evaluating the possibility of: (1) infectious diseases, (2) leukaemia, and (3) leucopenia due to certain psychotropic medications. This is particularly important for the monitoring of clozapine therapy (see below)
RBC count, Hemoglobin, Hematocrit	Important for evaluating polycythemia and anaemia, which may relate to a variety of psychotropics
Mean corpuscular volume (MCV)	Is the average volume of a RBC; useful in establishing whether an anaemia is macrocytic (ie, increased, such as in alcoholism, folate and B12 deficiency – often related to antiepileptic drugs (AEDs) or microcytic (i.e. decreased, such as in iron deficiency anaemia – sometimes related to NSAIDs)
Reticulocyte count	Gives an indication of RBC production and, hence, of bone marrow activity; increased in anaemias secondary to blood loss or hemolysis, decreased in anaemias secondary to impairment of RBC maturation (e.g. folate, B12 related to AEDs; iron deficiency anaemias before treatment)
Platelets	May be decreased due to drugs (e.g. valproate, phenothiazines) or due to medical illness; may occur along with other cell lines (pancytopenia)
Erythrocyte sedimentation rate (ESR)	A non-specific index of inflammation; elevated in infectious, neoplastic and inflammatory (e.g. vasculitis, systemic lupus erythematosus) illness
Coagulation tests	May be elevated in liver disease of many causes; Prothrombin time (PT), International normalized ratio (INR) used to monitor warfarin therapy; partial thromboplastin time (PTT) and activated partial thromboplastin time (APTT) used to monitor heparin therapy; need to be monitored closely in patients on warfarin taking psychotropics because of interactions (see section V)

RBC and serum folate; Vitamin B12 levels	Serum levels of folate and B12 used to screen for deficiency of these important vitamins; deficiency may present with or without concomitant anaemia with a variety of mental state changes (depression, psychosis, cognitive deficits, dementia) and/or neurological sequelae; deficiency may occur due to impaired absorption, deficient intake or secondary to medication (e.g. antiepileptic drugs); RBC folate should be monitored as it is more indicative of overall status than serum levels. The Schillings test and serum intrinsic factor are useful in evaluating B12 deficiency due to pernicious anaemia; it is important to monitor both B12 and folate as treatment with folate alone may reverse haematological abnormalities (macrocytic anaemia) without reversal of neurological deficits. Neurological and psychiatric manifestations of folate and B12 deficiency can occur with a normal haematological profile. Folate and B12 are affected by many drugs, particularly AEDs including phenytoin, carbamazepine and valproate. They should be measured in patients on these drugs as they are common contributors to psychiatric comorbidity and need to be supplemented appropriately. This is particularly important in women of child-bearing age where folate should be considered before conception (see section V for discussion of folate supplementation)
Thyroid Function Tests	Thyroid-stimulating hormone (TSH) is best screening test; serum triiodothyronine (T3), thyroxine (T4), reverse T3, T3 resin uptake (T3RU), free T4, free thyroxine index (FTI), antithyroglobulin antibodies and microsomal antibodies are also useful in the further evaluation of thyroid illness. Thyroid testing should be done to evaluate possible medication-induced thyroid disease (e.g. carbamazepine, lithium). Hypo- and hyper-thyroidism can present with a variety of psychiatric presentations, with improvement in mental state changes often lagging behind improvement in biochemical parameters. TFTs should be performed in all patients presenting with affective, psychotic or anxiety symptoms.
Dexamethasone Suppression Test (DST)	Measurement of serum cortisol checked at specific times before and after the administration of 1 mg dexamethasone, thought by some to be a biological marker for depression; a normal response, however, does not rule out the possibility of depression and an abnormal response must similarly be interpreted in the clinical context; may be useful in some ambiguous situations
Prolactin	Useful in evaluating patients on antipsychotics with galactorrhoea or to evaluate compliance, as antipsychotics characteristically increase prolactin; management of hyperprolactinaemia due to psychotropics is discussed in section VII; may be of limited use in evaluating nonepileptic seizure-like events (NESLEs) if psychotropics are controlled for and if sample is obtained within 20 minutes of a suspected seizure – a normal value, however, should not be interpreted as representing a NESLE, as no rise in levels may occur in seizures related to epilepsy as well. A clear rise in baseline within 20 min. of a seizure is useful as an indication of the seizure relating to epilepsy. Negative findings are of nebulous significance.

Laboratory tests and their relevance in psychiatry (*Continued*)

Electrolytes	Sodium (Na^+), potassium (K^+), chloride (Cl^-), and bicarbonate (HCO_3^-) are all useful screening tests in psychiatric illness and should also be monitored in patients on psychotropics (esp. carbamazepine and antidepressants) which may cause hyponatraemia; hyponatraemia is also seen in various medical illnesses and in SIADH and psychogenic polydipsia; hypokalaemia is common in people with bulimia and anorexia
Liver Function Tests	Useful screening test in psychiatric patients and also to be monitored in patients on psychotropics which may affect liver function (esp. antiepileptic drugs); includes alanine aminotransferase (ALT), alkaline phosphatase (AP), aspartate aminotransferase (AST), gamma-glutamyl transaminase (GGT) and lactate dehydrogenase (LDH) which has five isoenzymes and may be elevated in other medical conditions as well; GGT most sensitive of these; bilirubin (total, direct and indirect) useful in evaluation of hepatobiliary disease and haemolytic anaemia and may have to be ordered separately in some labs
Renal Function Tests	Blood urea nitrogen (BUN) and creatinine both elevated in renal failure; should be monitored in patients on lithium and amantadine
Amylase and lipase levels	Used to evaluate pancreatitis and pancreatic carcinoma; should be screened in patients on valproate with any gastrointestinal symptoms as this may induce pancreatitis; may also be a useful measure in monitoring bulimia
Glucose	Important test in evaluating both the possibility of diabetes mellitus as well as hypoglycaemia, which may present with a variety of intermittent mental state changes, including delirium and psychosis
Creatinine phosphokinase (CPK)	Useful in evaluating possible neuroleptic malignant syndrome (NMS) – see section VII for discussion
Copper and ceruloplasmin	Used to diagnose and evaluate Wilson's disease which is an inherited alteration in copper metabolism which presents with personality changes, altered cognition affective symptoms or psychosis associated with a movement disorder, usually in adolescents and young adults

Porphyrins	Porphobilinogen (PBG) aminolevulinic acid (ALA) and other porphyrins and metabolites used to diagnose porphyria, an inherited metabolic disorder which can present with intermittent psychosis and/or seizures or other neuropsychiatric manifestations; important as many psychotropics will exacerbate porphyria (see section V)
LE prep	Used along with other tests, including antinuclear antibodies (ANA), anti-DNA antibodies, lupus anticoagulant, and complement levels in the diagnosis of systemic lupus erythematosus (SLE); may present with depression, delirium, psychosis or dementia; phenothiazines, amongst other drugs, may cause false positives
RBC transketolase	Test for the diagnosis of Wernicke's encephalopathy (WE); WE is a medical emergency, commonly occurring in alcoholics and others deficient in thiamine; presents with mental status changes sometimes associated with opthalmoplegia / ataxia
Toxicology screens	Multiple drugs can be screened for at once; useful for suspected drug misuse and for suspected overdoses of an unknown substance; specific drugs may also be requested
Heavy metal screens	Many neuropsychiatric symptoms have been associated with lead, mercury, manganese, arsenic and aluminum poisoning; these should be tested if a patient with psychiatric presentation has any suggestion of a history of exposure to them

Plasma level monitoring of psychotropic and antiepileptic drugs

Monitoring plasma levels can assist in the overall treatment of the patient. However, blood tests are an inconvenience for both patients and staff, and drug assays add to laboratory time and costs. It is worthwhile knowing when and for which drugs plasma level monitoring is most useful. Situations when antiepileptic and psychotropic drug assays may be useful are:

✦ For monitoring patient concordance with drug therapy.

✦ For optimising the drug treatment of certain disorders where a target range has been identified e.g. phenytoin for epilepsy, lithium for prophylaxis of bipolar affective disorder.

✦ To confirm suspected toxicity, e.g. suspected lithium toxicity.

✦ In deciding when to start drug therapy after an intentional overdose, e.g. tricyclic anti-depressants.

✦ To confirm suspected drug interactions, or monitoring of potential drug interactions, e.g. using valproate and carbamazepine together.

✦ Monitoring drug levels in pregnancy and illness e.g. chronic liver disease.

✦ When treating patients who have difficulty in reporting adverse effects, e.g. children, patients with learning disabilities or cognitive impairment.

The drugs for which plasma level monitoring is most informative should fulfil all of the following criteria:

✦ There is an accurate and specific assay method available.

✦ There is a large variation in the excretion or metabolism of the drug between individual patients.

✦ The clinical response to the drug is difficult to assess.

✦ The difference in plasma level between the therapeutic level and the toxic level is small (i.e. narrow therapeutic index).

✦ The drug has no active metabolites.

Of the psychotropics and antiepileptics, lithium and phenytoin are the only drugs that fulfil this criteria. However, plasma level monitoring of drugs that fulfil some of these criteria can still be useful. See following table on page 10.

It is worth noting that when a "target range" for a drug is quoted, it is an *average* range in which most patients respond.

For example:

A patient taking carbamazepine for epilepsy has a carbamazepine level of 8mg/L (therapeutic range = 4–12mg/L). The patient does not experience any side-effects but is still having frequent seizures. Although the carbamazepine level is "in the range" it is prudent to increase the dose of carbamazepine in light of the lack of efficacy.

The time at which the blood sample is taken in relation to when the tablets are taken is vital for the plasma level to be meaningful. Even once the drug levels in the body are at steady-state (i.e. 4–5 × half-life after start of therapy), plasma levels vary throughout the day. Generally it is best to take blood samples when the plasma levels are lowest (i.e. a trough level), for example, taking pre-dose carbamazepine levels (see following table). After the first sample it is best for subsequent samples to be taken at the same time. Apparent variations in plasma levels are often the result of sampling at different times. In particular, the widespread practice of withholding doses until a sample is taken is especially likely to provide a spurious result. All results should be compared with previous values so that anomalies can be detected.

Plasma level monitoring of psychotropic and antiepileptic drugs

Drug	Sample time (time to steady state)	Recommended target concentration	Comments
Carbamazepine	pre-dose (1-2 weeks – see comments)	4-12 mg/L (epilepsy) 7-12 mg/L (bipolar affective disorder – see comments)	Active metabolite. Auto-induction occurs; wait 2 weeks after target dose is reached before sampling. Levels >7mg/L are thought to be associated with efficacy for mania and bipolar affective disorder (Taylor & Duncan, 1997).
Clozapine	pre-dose (2-4 days)	clozapine >350 mcg/L (> 0.35mg/L)	Perry et al (1991) showed that patients were more likely to respond if the plasma level was >350mcg/L (64% vs 22%) and that 5 of 7 non responders became responders when their level was increased to >350mcg/L. Similar results were found by Potkin et al, 1994. See also Taylor and Duncan (1995). Threshold may be as high as 500mcg/L – see section on clozapine.
Gabapentin	see comments	None	Plasma level monitoring is not currently recommended and the dose should be adjusted according to patient response.
Lamotrigine	see comments	None	Even though a recommended target concentration of 1-4mg/L has been suggested, a useful relationship has not been demonstrated between plasma concentration and effect or toxicity (Kilpatrick et al, 1996). The dose should be adjusted according to efficacy and tolerability.
Lithium	12 hours post-dose (5-7 days)	0.6-1.2 mmol/L	Plasma level monitoring should be done (minimum) weekly until target level reached, then monthly, then 3 monthly. Renal and thyroid function tests should be performed every six months.
Olanzapine	see comments	None	A therapeutic range has not yet been defined but an accurate and specific assay has been developed (Aravagiri et al, 1997).

Drug	Timing of sample	Therapeutic reference range	Comments
Phenobarbitone Primidone	pre-dose (2-3 weeks)	5-15 mg/L (primidone) 15-35 mg/L (phenobarbitone) 60-180 µmol/L (phenobarbitone)	As primidone is metabolised to phenobarbitone, it is essential to measure both levels in patients on primidone. Plasma levels may not be meaningful as tolerance develops.
Phenytoin	Pre-dose (2-14 days – dose dependent)	10-20 mg/L 40-80 µmols/L	Follows non-linear kinetics. Plasma level monitoring is essential. Highly protein bound, free levels are also useful, particularly at higher doses.
Valproate	pre-dose – at a fixed time in relation to meals – see comments (2-5 days)	50-100 mg/L (bipolar affective disorder)	Levels >50mg/L are thought to be effective for mania and bipolar affective disorder. No clear correlation for seizure control. Diurnal variation also affected by free fatty acid concentration in plasma. Highly protein bound, free levels are also useful (but rarely measured) especially at higher doses.
SSRIs	see comments	None	Plasma levels are not thought to be useful. Test compliance only.
Topiramate	see comments	None	No clear correlation between trough plasma concentrations and therapeutic response has been established.
Tricyclic antidepressants	see comments	Nortriptyline: 50-150 mcg/L (reference ranges for other tricyclics not as well established)	Most useful in suspected drug interactions or overdose and in people in whom there has been a poor response at normal doses.
Vigabatrin	see comments	None	No clear correlation between trough plasma concentrations and therapeutic response has been established.

Cerebrospinal fluid testing in psychiatry

Cerebrospinal fluid has many uses in psychiatry, but is predominantly used to rule out neurological disorders presenting with psychiatric symptoms. The following tables show the major indications and contraindications for this procedure.

Indications for lumbar puncture
modified from McConnell (1998) and McConnell and Bianchine (1994)

In adults:

❖ Suspected infections or post-infectious illness (bacterial, tuberculous viral and fungal meningitis, aseptic meningitis, infectious polyneuritis, HIV and herpes simplex encephalitis, encephalitis of uncertain cause)

❖ Multiple sclerosis (oligoclonal bands, IgG index and myelin basic protein most useful tests)

❖ Intracranial haemmorrhage (better evaluated in the first instance with neuroimaging; CSF may be diagnostic for subarachnoid haemmorrhage even if neuroimaging is negative, however)

❖ Meningeal malignancy (pleocytosis, – protein, – glucose, specific tumor markers)

❖ Paraneoplastic syndromes (specific neuronal nuclear and Purkinje cell antibodies detectable)

❖ Pseudotumor cerebri (requires lumbar puncture to diagnose)

❖ Normal pressure hydrocephalus

❖ Amyloid angiopathy (cystatin C, amyloid beta-protein)

❖ Neurosarcoidosis (CSF angiotensin converting enzyme)

❖ Evaluation of dementia (specific markers)

❖ Stroke (where CNS vasculitis is suspected, if septic emboli suspected, in patients with positive syphilis or HIV serology, and in young patients with unexplained strokes)

❖ Other (systemic lupus erythematosus, hepatic encephalopathy, vitamin B12 deficiency, occasionally in seizures to exclude CNS infection or bleed, and for intrathecal therapy)

In children:

❖ Suspected meningitis (CSF changes may be less specific and initially normal in children)

❖ Other infections (as with adults; most show non-specific changes except for antibody titers in SSPE, measles, rubella, and progressive rubella panencephalitis)

❖ Febrile seizures – only if clinical evidence of meningitis is present, except in infants <12 months where clinical signs may be absent and CSF should be examined)

❖ Intracranial haemmorhage in neonates

❖ Pseudotumor cerebri

❖ Lead encephalopathy

❖ CNS neoplasia (as with adults; best evaluated in the first instance with neuroimaging)

❖ Lysosomal storage diseases (measurement of specific glycosphingolipids)

❖ Therapeutic lumbar puncture (intrathecal therapy)

Contraindications to lumbar puncture
Modified from McConnell (1998) and McConnell and Bianchine (1994)

❖ If there is suspicion of increased intracranial pressure with a mass lesion or ventricular obstruction; in such instances neuroimaging should always be obtained first

❖ In the presence of complete spinal subarachnoid block

❖ In the presence of notable coagulation defects

❖ If there is evidence of local infection at the site of the lumbar puncture in the case of known bacteraemia, one should be extra careful with lumbar puncture as it has been associated with the occurrence of secondary meningitis

CSF levels of various psychotropics are readily measured but are of research interest only at this time. The interested reader is referred to McConnell (1998) and McConnell and Bianchine (1994).

Electroencephalography (EEG) in psychiatry

The EEG is a frequently used (and frequently misused!) tool in psychiatry. The table below shows the common indications for its use in treating patients with psychiatric illness.

Indications for EEG in psychiatry

Modified from McConnell (1998) and McConnell and Andrews (1999)

Indication	Comment
Suspected epilepsy	– Useful in the evaluation of episodic behavioural disorders e.g. atypical panic attacks, e.g. atypical paroxysmal affective or psychotic symptoms, rapid cycling, e.g. transient cognitive impairment or inattention in children – Sleep EEG and Ambulatory or video – EEG is often helpful – activation procedures are also useful – A normal EEG does not rule out epilepsy, nor does an abnormal EEG confirm it
Acute confusional states	– EEG is useful for both establishing the diagnosis and following the course of delirium
Other cognitive impairment	– EEG is useful in the diagnosis of dementia and of cognitive impairment related to depression or to medication effects
Other suspected neurological or medical illness presenting with psychiatric symptoms	– EEG indicated where findings in the history, mental state exam, physical exam or laboratory tests suggest a neurological or medical basis for the patient's symptoms **– EEG is not indicated for general screening of psychiatric patients or for the evaluation of primary psychiatric illness**
Electroconvulsive therapy (ECT)	– EEG monitoring useful to establish seizure duration during ECT
Suspected drug toxicity	– EEG is useful in evaluating suspected lithium and AED toxicity in patients who develop mental symptoms at therapeutic levels

The EEG is affected by many psychotropics and this must always be considered when ordering this test. These are summarised in the following table:

EEG changes related to treatment with psychotropics

Modified from McConnell and Andrews (1999) and McConnell and Snyder (1998)

Drug	Within therapeutic range	In overdose
Antipsychotics	– minor slowing of alpha – increased voltage of theta – clozapine may produce spike-wave complexes	– diffuse slowing – decreased alpha – occasionally increased sharp activity or spikes
Benzodiazepines	– increased beta activity	– diffuse slowing with superimposed beta activity
Lithium	– decreased amount and frequency of alpha activity	– diffuse slowing; decreased alpha; sharp waves
MAOIs	– usually none apparent	– diffuse slowing
SSRIs	– usually none apparent on visual inspection	– diffuse slowing – occasionally increased sharp activity or spikes
Stimulants	– increased beta and alpha activity	– diffuse slowing – sharp waves
Tricyclic antidepressants	– increased theta and/or beta activity – occasionally decreased alpha	– diffuse slowing – may be superimposed beta activity

15

References

American Psychiatric Association (1996) Practice Guidelines, APPress, Washington, DC., USA

Aravagiri M, Ames D, Wirshing WC, *et al* (1996) Plasma level monitoring of olanzapine in patients with schizophrenia: determination by high-performance liquid chromatography with electrochemical detection. *Therapeutic Drug Monitoring*, **19**, 307-313.

British Medical Association, Royal Pharmaceutical Society of Great Britain (1998) British National Formulary 36, *BMA / RPSGB*, London, U.K.

Ginestet D. (1996) Guide du Bon Usage des Psychotropes, Doin Editeurs, Paris, France

Kaplan HI, Sadock BJ. (1996) Pocket Handbook of Psychiatric Drug Treatment, American Psychiatric Press, Washington DC., U.S.A.

Kilpatrick ES, Forrest G, Brodie MJ. (1996) Concentration-effect and concentration-toxicity relations with lamotrigine: a prospective study. *Epilepsia*, **37,** 534-538.

McConnell H. (1998) Psychological and Behavioral Correlates of Blood and CSF Laboratory Tests. In: PJ Snyder & PD Nussbaum (Eds), Clinical Neuropsychology for House Staff, American Psychological Press, Washington, U.S.A.

McConnell H, Bianchine J. (1994) Cerebrospinal Fluid in Neurology and Psychiatry. Chapman Hall, London, U.K.

McConnell H, Andrews C. (1999) The EEG in Psychiatry. In: *Clinical Neurophysiology*. C. Binnie (ed), Blackwell, Oxford, U.K.

McConnell H, Snyder PJ. (1998) Electroencephalography in the elderly. In: P.Nussbaum (Ed.), Handbook of Neuropsychology and Aging. A volume in the *Critical Issues in Neuropsychology* series (E.E. Puente & C.R. Reynolds, Eds.). New York: Plenum Press.

Perry PJ, Miller DD, Arndt SV, *et al* (1991) Clozapine and norclozapine plasma concentrations and clinical response of treatment refractory schizophrenic patients. *American Journal of Psychiatry*, **148**, 231-235.

Potkin SG, Bera R, Gulasekaram B, *et al* (1994) Plasma clozapine concentrations predict clinical response in treatment-resistant schizophrenia. *Journal of Clinical Psychiatry*, **55** (Suppl. 9B), 133-136.

Rosse RB, Giese A, Deutsch S, Morihisa JM (1989) Laboratory Diagnostic Testing in Psychiatry, American Psychiatric Press, Washington DC, U.S.A.

Smith P, Darlington C. (1996) Clinical Psychopharmacology. Lawrence Erlbaum Associates, Mahwah, NJ, U.S.A.

Snyder PJ and McConnell H. (1998) Epilepsy in the Elderly. In: P. Nussbaum (Ed.) Handbook of Neuropsychology and Aging. A volume in the *Critical Issues in Neuropsychology* series (A.E. Puente & C.R. Reynolds, Eds.). Plenum Press, New York, U.S.A.

Taylor DM, Duncan D. (1995). The use of clozapine plasma levels in optimising therapy. *Psychiatric Bulletin,* **19**, 753-755.

Taylor D, Duncan D. (1997) Doses of carbamazepine and valproate in bipolar affective disorder. *Psychiatric Bulletin,* **21**, 221-223.

Taylor D, Paton C. (1998) Case studies in Psychopharmacolgy: The Use of Drugs in Psychiatry, Martin Dunitz, London, U.K.

Victorian Drug Usage Advisory Committee (1995) Psychotropic Drug Guidelines, VMPF Therapeutics Committee, Victoria, Australia.

| Drug | Obligatory monitoring | | Suggested additional |
	Baseline	Continuation	Baseline
Amisulpride	None	None	CPK FBC Prolactin U&Es Weight
Clozapine	FBC Prescriber and pharmacist must register	FBC – weekly for 18 wks – at least every 2 wks for 1 year – monthly thereafter	Blood glucose BP CPK ECG EEG LFTs V&Es Weight
Olanzapine	None	None	Blood glucose BP CPK FBC LFTs U&Es Prolactin Weight
Quetiapine	None	None	Blood glucose BP CPK FBC LFTs TFTs U&Es Weight
Risperidone	None	None	BP CPK FBC LFTs Prolactin U&Es Weight
Zotepine	None	None	Blood glucose BP CPK EEG ECG FBC LFTs Prolactin U&Es Weight

KEY:

–BP	Blood Pressure	–CPK	Creatinine Phosphokinase
–FBC	Full blood count	–LFTs	Liver function tests
–U&Es	Urea & electrolytes		

suggested monitoring

monitoring		Actions
Continuation		
CPK	– if NMS suspected	Stop if NMS suspected
FBC	– 6 monthly	Stop if neutrophils below 1.5 × 10⁹/L
Prolactin	– if symptoms occur	Stop if prolactin-related effects intolerable
U&Es	– 6 monthly	
Weight	– as needed	
Blood glucose [1,2]	– 3–6 monthly	Stop if NMS suspected
BP	– 4 hourly during titration	Stop if neutrophils below 1.5 × 10⁹/L
CPK	– if NMS suspected	Refer to specialist care if neutrophils below 0.5 × 10⁹/L
ECG [3,4]	– when maintenance dose is reached	Stop if ECG shows important changes or if signs of heart failure noted
EEG [5,6]	– if myoclonus or seizures occur	Stop if LFTs indicate hepatitis or reduced hepatic function (PT)
LFTs [7]	– every 3–6 months	Use valproate if EEG shows epileptiform changes
U&Es [8]	– every 6 months	
Weight	– as needed	
Blood glucose [1,9,10]	– 3–6 monthly	Stop if NMS suspected
BP	– frequently during initiation	Stop if neutrophils below 1.5 × 10⁹/L
CPK	– if NMS suspected	Stop if PT or bilirubin change
FBC [11]	– 3–6 monthly	
LFTs	– monthly for 3 months	
U&Es	– 6 monthly	
Prolactin	– if symptoms occur (rare)	
Weight	– as needed	
Blood glucose [12]	– 3–6 monthly	Stop if NMS suspected
BP	– frequently during titration	Stop if neutrophils below 1.5 × 10⁹/L
CPK	– if NMS suspected	Stop if PT or bilirubin change
FBC	– 3–6 monthly	
LFTs	– monthly for 3 months	
TFTs	– 6 monthly	
U&Es	– 6 monthly	
Weight	– as needed	
BP	– frequently during titration	Stop if NMS suspected
CPK	– if NMS suspected	Stop if neutrophils below 1.5 × 10⁹/L
FBC	– 3–6 monthly	Stop if prolactin-related effects intolerable
LFTs	– 3–6 monthly	Use with caution in hepatic/renal failure
Prolactin	– if symptoms occur	
U&Es	– 6 monthly	
Weight	– as needed	
Blood glucose	– 3–6 monthly	Stop if NMS suspected
BP	– frequently during titration	Stop if neutrophils below 1.5 × 10⁹/L
CPK	– if NMS suspected	Use valproate if EEG shows epileptiform changes
EEG [13]	– if seizures occur	Stop if ECG shows important changes
ECG	– when maintenance dose is reached	Stop if renal function deteriorates
FBC	– 3–6 monthly	
LFTs	– 3–6 monthly	
Prolactin	– if symptoms occur	
U&Es	– 6 monthly	
Weight	– as needed	

–ECG	Electrocardiograph	–EEG	Electro–encephalograph
–PT	Prothrombin time	–TFTs	Thyroid Function Tests

New antipsychotics – suggested monitoring

Sources of information

Monitoring recommendations for new antipsychotics are derived from:

i)   Normal clinical practice with new medicines (e.g. FBC, LFTs, U&Es).
ii) Relevant summaries of product characteristics.
iii) Specific references below.

References

1. Wirshing DA, Spellberg BJ, Erhart SM, *et al.* (1998) Novel antipsychotics and new onset diabetes. *Biol Psychiatry*, **44**, 778–783.
2. Hägg S, Joelsson L, Mjörndal T, *et al.* (1998) Prevalence of diabetes and impaired glucose tolerance in patients treated with clozapine compared with patients treated with conventional depot neuroleptic medications. *J Clin Psychiatry*, **59**, 294–299.
3. Leo RJ, Kreeger JL, Kim KY. (1996) Cardiomyopathy associated with clozapine. *Ann Pharmacother*, **30**, 603–605.
4. Low RA, Fuller MA, Popli A. (1998) Clozapine induced atrial fibrillation. *Clin Psychopharmacol*, **18**, 170 (Letter).
5. Silvestri RC, Bromfield EB, Khoshbin S. (1998) Clozapine-induced seizures and EEG abnormalities in ambulatory psychiatric patients. *Ann Pharmacother*, **32**, 1147–1151.
6. Taner E, Cosar B, Isik E. (1998) Clozapine-induced myoclonic seizures and valproic acid. *Int J Psych Clin Prac*, **2**, 53–55.
7. Hummer M, Kurz M, Kurzthaler I, *et al.* (1997) Hepatotoxicity of clozapine. *J Clin Psychopharmacol*, **17**, 314–317.
8. Elias TJ, Bannister KM, Clarkson AR, *et al.* (1999) Clozapine: First report of acute interstitial nephritis: case report. *Lancet*, **354**, 1180–1.
9. Ober SK, Hudak R, Rusterholtz A. (1999) Hyperglycemia and olanzapine. *Am J Psychiatry*, **156**, 970.
10. Lindenmayer JP, Patel R. (1999) Olanzapine-induced ketoacidosis with diabetes mellitus. *Am J Psychiatry*, **156**, 1471.
11. Naumann R, Felber W, Heilemann H, *et al.* (1999) Olanzapine-induced agranulocytosis. *Lancet*, **354**, 566–567.
12. Sobel M, Jaggers ED, Franz MA. (1999) New-onset diabetes mellitus associated with the initiation of quetiapine treatment. *J Clin Psychiatry*, **60**, 556–557.
13. Prakash A, Lamb HM. (1998) Zotepine: a review of its pharmacodynamic and pharmacokinetic properties and therapeutic efficacy in the management of schizophrenia. *CNS Drugs*, **Feb: 9**, 153–175.

Further Reading

Taylor D. (1997) Monitoring the new antipsychotic drugs. *Progress in Neurology and Psychiatry*, **1**, 13–15.

II

Treatment of

Psychosis

Antipsychotics – general principles of prescribing

Aims

To ensure quality of prescribing of all antipsychotics and to shift the spectrum of use of novel antipsychotics from difficult to treat patients (for which only clozapine is indicated) to patients in earlier phases of illness.

Standards

✦ Each patient should ideally be prescribed only one antipsychotic, preferably in a single dosage form. (An exception is when switching from one drug to another.)

✦ Typical antipsychotics should ideally not be used as "PRN" sedatives. (Short courses of benzodiazepines or general sedatives (e.g. promethazine) may be used.)

✦ The lowest possible effective dose should be used, with patients given a sufficient trial on low doses before any further dose increases. This applies to both typical and atypical antipsychotics.

✦ *As a consequence,* doses above 15mg/day haloperidol or equivalent should be the exception rather than the rule. Patients receiving higher doses without resolution of symptoms should be considered for clozapine.

✦ Patients receiving >1g equivalent chlorpromazine should be monitored as outlined by the Royal College of Psychiatrists. Those showing a measured response should have this documented in their notes. Those not responding should be considered for clozapine.

✦ Anticholinergic drugs should be given for Parkinsonism or dystonia (prophylactically as necessary) but withdrawal should be attempted after 2–3 months without symptoms. Anticholinergics are liable to misuse and impair memory.

✦ Individual *atypical* antipsychotics should be used for the indications outlined on page 34.

✦ Standard clinical rating scales should be used to evaluate changes in symptoms.

Drug	Chemical group	Dose range (daily dose) Single daily dose unless stated (*)	Alternative indications
Chlorpromazine	Phenothiazine (Grp I – aliphatic)	25–1000mg	Anxiety, nausea, agitation, hiccup, induction of hypothermia, violence, autism
Promazine	Phenothiazine (Grp I – aliphatic)	400–800mg	Agitation and restlessness in the elderly. **NB.** Weak antipsychotic
Thioridazine	Phenothiazine (Grp II – piperidine)	150–800mg	Agitation, anxiety, violence, impulsive behaviour. Agitation and restlessness in the elderly
Fluphenazine	Phenothiazine (Grp III – piperazine)	1–20mg	Agitation, anxiety, violence
Perphenazine	Phenothiazine (Grp III – piperazine)	12–24mg	Agitation, severe anxiety, violence
Trifluoperazine	Phenothiazine (Grp III – piperazine)	10–50mg (est.) (maximum dose not stated by manufacturers)	Agitation, severe anxiety, violence
Flupenthixol	Thioxanthine	6–18mg	Depressive illness (lower doses)
Zuclopenthixol	Thioxanthine	20–150mg	None
Haloperidol	Butyrophenone	1.5–120mg	Agitation, severe anxiety, violence, tics, nausea, hiccup, mania, Gilles de la Tourette
Droperidol	Butyrophenone	20–120mg (*QDS)	Anaesthesia, mania, nausea. **NB.** For acute (sedative) treatment only
Benperidol	Butyrophenone	0.25–1.5mg (*BD)	Deviant social/sexual behaviour. **NB.** Not licensed for schizophrenia

Adverse effects (See data sheet for full details/section VII for comparison)	Interactions (See manufacturers' data for full information)	Cost
Extrapyramidal effects, anticholinergic effects, sedation, hypotension, hypothermia, endocrine disorders, convulsions, jaundice, ECG changes, blood dyscrasias	Sedatives, lithium, anticholinergics, antiepileptics, sulphonylureas, cimetidine, antidepressants, dopamine (ant)agonists	+
As chlorpromazine	As chlorpromazine	+
As chlorpromazine + pigmented retinopathy, ejaculatory dysfunction	As chlorpromazine	+
As chlorpromazine + depression reported	As chlorpromazine	+
As chlorpromazine	As chlorpromazine	+
As chlorpromazine	As chlorpromazine	+
As chlorpromazine	As chlorpromazine	+
As chlorpromazine	As chlorpromazine	+
As chlorpromazine	As chlorpromazine + fluoxetine, carbamazepine, astemizole, terfenadine	+
As chlorpromazine + depression	As chlorpromazine	++
As chlorpromazine	As chlorpromazine	++

Drug	Chemical group	Dose range (daily dose) Single daily dose unless stated (*)	Alternative indications
Sulpiride	Substituted benzamide	400–2400mg (*BD)	None
Pimozide	Diphenylbutylpiperidine	2–20mg	Mania, hypochondriacal psychosis
Loxapine	Dibenzoxazepine	20–250mg (*BD)	None
Risperidone	Benzisoxazole	2–16mg	None
Olanzapine	Thienobenzodiazepine	5–20 mg/day	None
Quetiapine	Dibenzothiazepine	150–750mg (*BD) Lower doses in the elderly	None
Amisulpride	Substituted benzamide	Positive symptoms 400–1200mg (*BD) Negative Symptoms: 50–300mg	None
Ziprasidone (not licensed in UK at time of publication)	Benzothiazolylpiperazine	40–160mg/day (*BD)	None
Zotepine	Dibenzothiepine	50–300mg/day (*TDS)	None
Clozapine **See data sheet for restrictions to licence**	Dibenzodiazepine	25–900mg (*BD or more frequently)	None

Adverse effects (See data sheet for full details/section VII for comparison)	Interactions (See manufacturers' data for full information)	Cost
As chlorpromazine, jaundice & skin reactions less common. Less sedation, hypotension	As chlorpromazine	++
As chlorpromazine + serious cardiac arrhythmias (monitor plasma potassium), depression	As chlorpromazine + diuretics, any cardioactive drug – this includes other antipsychotics and tricyclics	+
As chlorpromazine + nausea, dyspnoea, ptosis, polydipsia, paraesthesia	As chlorpromazine	++
Agitation, hypotension, abdominal pain, fatigue, anxiety, nausea, rhinitis, weight gain, etc. EPS uncommon with doses below 8mg/day. Prolactin changes may cause sexual dysfunction, etc	As chlorpromazine	+++
Sedation, weight gain, hypotension, anticholinergic effects, changes in LFTs	Smoking and carbamazepine reduce olanzapine levels to small extent	+++
Hypotension, sedation, dry mouth, constipation, weight gain, dizziness, LFT changes, TFT changes	Caution with potent inhibitors of CYP3A4. (e.g. ketoconazole/nefazodone)	+++
Insomnia, agitation, anxiety, weight gain, extrapyramidal adverse effects, hyper-prolactinaemia, sedation	Few known interactions. Caution with other sedatives, including alcohol; dopamine agonists; and possibly hypotensives	+++
Somnolence, nausea Rarely – dystonia, postural hypotension	Few known interactions – does not inhibit cytochrome enzymes. Ziprasidone levels slightly ↓ by carbamazepine and ↑ by cimetidine	+++?
As chlorpromazine + creatinine increase; hypouricaemia	As chlorpromazine + zotepine levels increased by CYP3A4 inhibitors such as diazepam and fluoxetine	++
As chlorpromazine + hypersalivation, delirium, incontinence, myocarditis, neutropenia, fatal agranulocytosis (see table)	As chlorpromazine + all drugs which depress leucopoiesis: eg cytotoxic agents, sulphonamides, chloramphenicol, carbamazepine, phenothiazines. SSRIs (not citalopram) and risperidone increase clozapine plasma levels. Smoking, carbamazepine and phenytoin decrease clozapine levels	++++

Schizophrenia and psychosis in primary care – golden rules for prescribing

✦ **If in doubt about diagnosis, refer to specialist immediately.** The longer the period of untreated psychosis, the worse the prognosis.

✦ **Prescribe <u>one</u> antipsychotic at a time.** Avoid polypharmacy, particularly of typicals and atypicals in combination.

✦ **Encourage dialogue with patients in regard to acceptability of drug treatment.** Preferable alternatives can usually be found.

✦ **Monitor treatment.** Do this in accordance with suggested scheme on pages 18–20, or as agreed in local shared-care programme.

Drug treatment of schizophrenia

Atypical antipsychotics
Summary of recommendations

Atypical antipsychotics are recommended as:

✦ 1st line therapy in first episode schizophrenia.

✦ Alternatives to typical drugs in patients suffering intolerable or dangerous adverse effects on typicals.

✦ Treatment for refractory schizophrenia (clozapine only).

Treatment of schizophrenia

1st episode schizophrenic psychosis – protocol

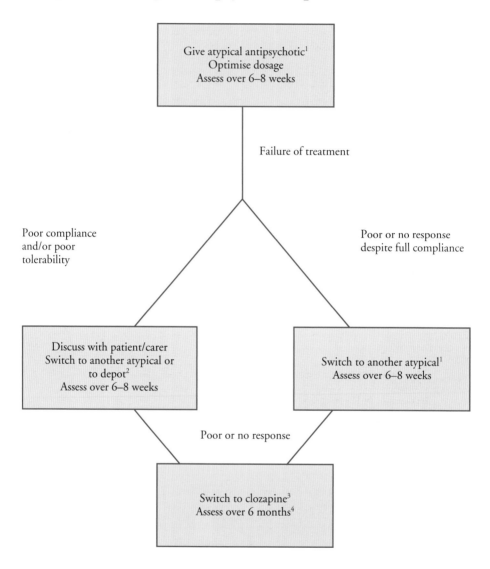

Give atypical antipsychotic[1]
Optimise dosage
Assess over 6–8 weeks

Failure of treatment

Poor compliance and/or poor tolerability

Poor or no response despite full compliance

Discuss with patient/carer
Switch to another atypical or to depot[2]
Assess over 6–8 weeks

Switch to another atypical[1]
Assess over 6–8 weeks

Poor or no response

Switch to clozapine[3]
Assess over 6 months[4]

1st episode schizophrenia – notes

	Notes	References
1.	Atypicals are recommended first line on the basis that they are better tolerated than typical drugs at normal clinical doses. Specifically, all atypicals cause less severe extrapyramidal effects than haloperidol. Quetiapine and perhaps olanzapine seem to cause no more extrapyramidal effects than placebo Symptomatic hyperprolactinaemia seems not to occur with quetiapine or olanzapine.	Mir S, Taylor D. (1998) Schizophrenia. *Pharm Journal*, **261**, 55–58. Arvanitis LA, Miller BG. *(1997)* Multiple fixed doses of "Seroquel" (quetiapine) in patients with acute exacerbation of schizophrenia: a comparison with haloperidol and placebo. *Biol Psychiatry*, **42**, 233–246. Tran PV, Dellva MA, Tollefson GD, *et al.* (1997) Extrapyramidal symptoms and tolerability of olanzapine versus haloperidol in the acute treatment of schizophrenia. *J Clin Psychiatry*, **58**, 205–211. Hamner MB, Arana GW. (1998) Hyperprolactinaemia in antipsychotic-treated patients: guidelines for and management. *CNS Drugs*, **10**, 209–222.
	Tardive dyskinesia is less frequent with olanzapine than with haloperidol. Less compelling data with other atypicals but reduced acute extra-pyramidal effects may portend lower rates of TD.	Tollefson GD, Beasley CM, Tamura RN, *et al.* (1997) Double-blind, controlled, long-term study of the comparative incidence of treatment-emergent tardive dyskinesia with olanzapine or haloperidol. *Am J Psychiatry*, **154**, 1248–1254. Beasley CM, Dellva MA, Tamura RN, *et al.* (1999) Randomised double-blind comparison of the incidence of tardive dyskinesia in patients with schizophrenia during long-term treatment with olanzapine or haloperidol. *Br J Psychiatry*, **174**, 23–30.
	There is some evidence that olanzapine is more effective than haloperidol in 1st episode psychosis.	Sanger TM, Lieberman JA, Tohen M, *et al.* (1999) Olanzapine versus haloperidol treatment in first-episode psychosis. *Am J Psychiatry*, **156**, 79–87.
	"Low dose" typical drugs cannot be recommended as an alternative to atypical drugs. Extrapyramidal side effects, symptomatic hyperprolactinaemia and tardive dyskinesia all appear at doses too low to be uniformly therapeutic.	Zimbroff DL, Kane JM, Tamminga CA *et al.* (1997) Controlled, dose-response study of sertindole and haloperidol in the treatment of schizophrenia. *Am J Psychiatry*, **154**, 783–791. Jeste DV, Lacro JP, Palmer B, *et al.* *(1999)* Incidence of tardive dyskinesia in early stages of low-dose treatment with typical neuroleptics in older patients. *Am J Psychiatry*, **156**, 309–311. Meltzer HY, Fang VS. (1976) The effect of neuroleptics on serum prolactin in schizophrenic patients. *Arch Gen Psychiatry*, **33**, 279–286.
	Sulpiride is essentially typical.	Caley CF, Weber SS. (1995) Sulpiride: an antipsychotic with selective dopaminergic antagonist properties. *Ann Pharmacother*, **29**, 152–160.

	Notes	References
2.	Typical depots reduce relapse and re-hospitalisation Atypical depots, when available, are likely to be preferred treatment.	Davis JM, Matalon L, Watanabe MD, *et al.* (1994) Depot antipsychotic drugs: place in therapy. *Drugs,* **47**, 741–773.
3.	Only clozapine has proven efficacy in treatment-refractory schizophrenia. Time taken to receive effective treatment is a powerful prognostic indicator. Search for effective treatment is therefore a matter of urgency. Clozapine treatment should not be delayed.	Taylor D. (1999) Refractory schizophrenia: evidence-based treatment. *Pharm Journal,* **263** (Suppl 1), 2–3. Launer M, MacKeen W. (2000) Effective management of schizophrenia within primary care. *Progress in Neurology and Psychiatry,* **3**, 24–27. Kasper S. (1999) First episode schizophrenia: the importance of early intervention and subjective tolerability. *J Clin Psychiatry,* **60**, [Suppl 23]; 5–9. Loebel AB, Lieberman JA, Alvir JMJ, *et al.* (1992) Duration of psychosis and outcome in first-episode schizophrenia. *Am J Psychiatry,* **149**, 1183–1188.
4.	Some debate surrounds the appropriate time period of evaluation. Most responders can be identified within 3 months but a substantial minority meet criteria for response after 3–12 months.	Carpenter WT, Conley RR, Buchanan RW, *et al.* (1995) Patient response and resource management: another view of clozapine treatment of schizophrenia. *Am J Psychiatry,* **152**, 827–832. Wilson, WH. (1996) Time required for initial improvement during clozapine treatment of refractory schizophrenia. *Am J Psychiatry,* **153**, 951–952.

Relapse or acute exacerbation of schizophrenia

Full adherence to medication confirmed

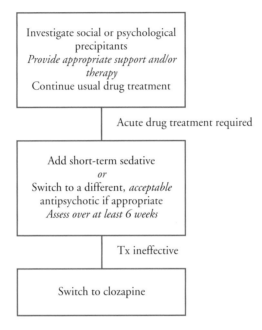

Investigate social or psychological precipitants
Provide appropriate support and/or therapy
Continue usual drug treatment

Acute drug treatment required

Add short-term sedative
or
Switch to a different, *acceptable* antipsychotic if appropriate
Assess over at least 6 weeks

Tx ineffective

Switch to clozapine

Adherence doubtful or known to be poor

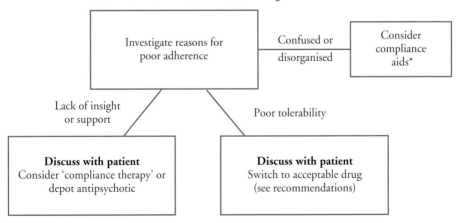

Investigate reasons for poor adherence

Confused or disorganised

Consider compliance aids*

Lack of insight or support

Poor tolerability

Discuss with patient
Consider 'compliance therapy' or depot antipsychotic

Discuss with patient
Switch to acceptable drug (see recommendations)

* Compliance aids (e.g. Medidose system) are not a substitute for patient education. The aim should be to promote independent living, perhaps with the patient filling their own compliance aid, having first been given support and training.

Switching drugs – recommendations

◆ **Extrapyramidal effects (including secondary negative symptoms)**
Switch to quetiapine[1] or olanzapine.[1] Low dose (4mg/day) risperidone also an option[1,2]

◆ **Hyperprolactinaemia**
Switch to quetiapine[3] or olanzapine.[3,4]

◆ **Weight gain**
Provide advice and support on healthy eating and exercise. Consider switching drug to one less likely to cause weight gain (e.g. (see page 199) amisulpride, sulpiride or ziprasidone, where available, may be appropriate).[5] In severe cases, refer to specialist.

◆ **Sedation**
Lower dose. Switch to less sedative drug (risperidone, amisulpride, haloperidol, etc.)

◆ **Tardive dyskinesia**
Switch to clozapine[6] or (possibly) olanzapine,[7,8] or (perhaps) quetiapine.[9]

◆ **Postural hypotension**
Switch to amisulpride. Consider also sulpiride, haloperidol and trifluoperazine.

References

1. Stanniland C, Taylor D. (2000) Tolerability of atypical antipsychotics. *Drug Saf*, **22**, 195–214.
2. Lemmens P, Brecher M, Van Baelen B. (1999) A combined analysis of double-blind studies with risperidone vs. placebo and other antipsychotic agents: factors associated with extrapyramidal symptoms. *Acta Psychiatr Scand*, **99**, 160–170.
3. Hammer MB, Arana GW. (1998) Hyperprolactinaemia in antipsychotic-treated patients: guidelines for avoidance and management. *CNS Drugs*, **10**, 209–222.
4. Rapid reduction in hyperprolactinemia upon switching treatment to olanzapine from conventional antipsychotic drugs or risperidone. Poster presented at American Psychiatric Association annual meeting, May 2000, Chicago, Illinois.
5. Taylor DM, McAskill R. (2000) Atypical antipsychotics and weight gain—a systematic review. *Acta Psychiatr Scand*, **101**, 416–432.
6. Lieberman J, Johns C, Cooper T, *et al.* (1989) Clozapine pharmacology and tardive dyskinesia. *Psychopharmacology*, **99**, S54–S59.
7. O'Brien J, Barber R. (1998) Marked improvement in tardive dyskinesia following treatment with olanzapine in an elderly subject. *Br J Psychiatry*, **172**, 186 (Letter).
8. Kinon BJ, Milton DR, Stauffer VL, *et al.* Effect of chronic olanzapine treatment on the course of presumptive tardive dyskinesia. Poster presented at American Psychiatric Association 152nd Annual Meeting, May 1999, Washington, DC.
9. Reznik I, Benatov R, Sirota P. (2000) Long-term efficacy and safety of quetiapine in treatment-refractory schizophrenia: a case report. *Int J Psych Clin Prac*, **4**, 77–80.

Prescribing in schizophrenia – use of typical antipsychotics

Typical antipsychotics have been widely used for nearly 50 years. They are cheap and much is known about their therapeutic and adverse effects. However, acute extrapyramidal effects, hyperprolactinaemia and tardive dyskinesia are well-known consequences of the use of typical drugs. Moreover there is essentially no evidence to suggest that using low doses of typical drugs reduces adverse effect burden: all typical adverse effects seem to occur at doses too low to produce therapeutic effects (see protocol for 1st episode psychosis). Note also that prophylaxis with anticholinergic drugs is only partly effective at preventing movement disorder,[1] and that anticholinergics are likely to worsen cognitive deficits seen in schizophrenia.

Typical antipsychotics are rarely recommended in protocols in this edition of the *Maudsley Prescribing Guidelines*. Two notable exceptions are the use of depots in those known to be poor compliers with medication and the use of parenteral typicals in rapid tranquillisation. In both cases, typical therapy is likely to be eventually superceded, by, respectively, risperidone depot, and olanzapine and ziprasidone intramuscular preparations, assuming these do become available and their use is cogently supported by published data.

It is recognised that many patients are stabilised on typical therapy and that many clinicians will feel it unwise to change medication in such patients. Continuation may be appropriate, for example, where typicals are effective and well tolerated, but the risk of tardive dyskinesia should be borne in mind. Perhaps more importantly, the funding of atypical antipsychotics is highly variable. This often means that the prescribing of atypicals is at least partly restricted by the absence of necessary funding.[2] It should also be noted that some people tolerate typical drugs very well and in some cases may prefer them to atypicals.

Where typicals continue to be used for whatever reason, minimisation of risk is of great importance. Below, we discuss some possible therapeutic options for risk minimisation.

Acute extrapyramidal adverse effects

Typicals vary somewhat in their propensity to cause acute movement disorders.

Thioridazine has intrinsic anticholinergic activity which probably reduces the frequency and severity of acute movement disorders. However, because of its profound anticholinergic effects it is often poorly tolerated and it is well known to affect adversely cardiac rhythm,[3] cause retinopathy[4] and hyperprolactinaemia is induced by as little as 200mg/day.[5]

Pimozide may also cause less severe or frequent acute movement disorders but it too is cardio-toxic and induces hyperprolactinaemia at 6mg/day.[6] It is now only rarely prescribed.

Sulpiride is only weakly associated with lower rates of acute movement disorders.[7] Hyperprolactinaemia is very common and often symptomatic.

Hyperprolactinaemia

All typical agents appear to cause significant rises in serum prolactin which can lead to a range of unpleasant or disturbing adverse events. Although not widely investigated, it seems that typicals engender hyperprolactinaemia at doses substantially below those required for therapeutic efficacy.[8]

Tardive dyskinesia (TD)

The incidence of TD observed with typical drugs is 5% year on year, with a prevalence of around 25%.[9] No one typical agent has been conclusively shown to have any advantage in this regard. The emergence of early extrapyramidal effects seems to be a compelling risk factor for later TD but data on the influence of antipsychotic doses are equivocal.[9,10] Despite this latter observation it seems intuitively to be prudent to keep the dose of typical drugs low and to avoid polypharmacy.

References

1. Keepers G, Clappison V, Casey D. (1983) Initial anticholinergic prophylaxis for neuroleptic-induced extrapyramidal syndromes. *Arch Gen Psychiatry,* **40,** 1113–1117.
2 Taylor D, Mir S, Mace S, *et al.* (1999) Is cost a factor (ii)? The National Schizophrenia Fellowship.
3. Simpson G, Pi E, Sramek J. (1981) Adverse effects of antipsychotic agents. *Drugs,* **21,** 138–151.
4. Tekell J, Silva J, Maas, J, *et al.* (1996) Thioridazine-induced retinopathy. *Am J Psychiatry,* **153:9,** 1234–1235.
5. Meltzer H, Fang V. (1976) The effect of neuroleptics on serum prolactin in schizophrenic patients. *Arch Gen Psychiatry,* **33,** 279–286.
6. Nishikawa T, Tsuda A, Tanaka M, *et al.* (1985) Prophylactic effects of neuroleptics in symptom-free schizophrenics: roles of dopaminergic and noradrenergic blockers. *Biol Psychiatry,* **20,** 1161–1166.
7. Caley C, Weber S. (1995) Sulpiride: an antipsychotic with selective dopaminergic antagonist properties. *Ann Pharmacother,* **29,** 152–160.
8. Hamner B, Arana W. (1998) Hyperprolactinaemia in antipsychotic-treated patients: guidelines for avoidance and management. *CNS Drugs,* **10(3),** 209–222.
9. Jeste D, Caligiuri M. (1993) Tardive dyskinesia. *Schizophr Bull,* **19(2),** 303–315.
10. Cavallaro R, Smeraldi E. (1995) Antipsychotic-induced tardive dyskinesia: recognition, prevention and management. *CNS Drugs,* **4(4),** 278–293.

Optimising clozapine treatment

Target dose *(Note that dose is best adjusted according to patient tolerability)*	❖ Average dose in UK is around 450mg/day	Taylor D, Mace S, Mir S, Kerwin R. (2000) A prescription survey of the use of atypical antipsychotics for hospital inpatients in the United Kingdom. *Int J Psych in Clin Prac,* **4**, 41–46.
	❖ Response usually seen in the range 150–900mg/day	Murphy B, Long C, Paton C. (1998) Maintenance doses for clozapine. *Psych Bull,* **22**, 12–14.
	❖ Lower doses required in the elderly, females and non-smokers, and in those prescribed certain enzyme inhibitors	Taylor D. (1997) Pharmacokinetic interactions involving clozapine. *Br J Psychiatry,* **171**, 109–112. Lane HY, Chang YC, Chang WH, *et al.* (1999) Effects of gender and age on plasma levels of clozapine and its metabolites: analysed by critical statistics. *J Clin Psychiatry,* **60**, 36–40.
Plasma levels	Most studies indicate that threshold for response is in the range 350–420mcg/L Threshold may be as high as 500mcg/L Importance of nor-clozapine levels not established	Taylor D, Duncan D. (1995) The use of clozapine plasma levels in optimising therapy. *Psych Bull,* **19**, 753–755. Spina E, Avenoso A, Facciolà G, *et al.* (2000) Relationship between plasma concentrations of clozapine and norclozapine and therapeutic response in patients with schizophrenia resistant to conventional neuroleptics. *Psychopharmacol,* **148**, 83–89. Perry PJ. (2000) Therapeutic drug monitoring of atypical antipsychotics: Is it of potential clinical value? *CNS Drugs,* **13**, 167–171.

Optimising clozapine treatment

Other suggested options where 3–6 months of clozapine alone has provided no clear benefit:

Add sulpiride (400mg/day)	❖ May be useful in partial or non-responders	Shiloh R, Zemishlany Z, Aizenberg D, *et al.* (1997) Sulpiride augmentation in people with schizophrenia partially responsive to clozapine. *B J Psychiatry*, **171**, 569–573.
Add lamotrigine (25–200mg/day)	❖ As sulpiride	Dursun SM, McIntosh D. (1999) Clozapine plus lamotrigine in treatment-resistant schizophrenia. *Arch Gen Psychiatry*, **56**, 950.
Add risperidone (2mg/day)	❖ Increases clozapine plasma levels May have additive effects	Morera AL, Barreiro P, Cano-Muñoz JL. (1999) Case report: Risperidone and clozapine combination for the treatment of refractory schizophrenia. *Acta Psych Scand* **99**, 305–307. Raskin S, Katz G, Zislin Z, *et al.* (2000) Clozapine and risperidone: combination/augmentation treatment of refractory schizophrenia: a preliminary observation. *Acta Psych Scan*, **101**, 334–336.
Add **omega-3-triglycerides** (Maxepa 5G BD)	❖ Modest, if contested, evidence that Maxepa gives improvement in non- or partial responders to antipsychotics	McGorry PD, Yung AR, Phillips L, *et al.* (1998) Double-blind placebo controlled trial of N-3 polyunsaturated fatty acids as an adjunct to neuroleptics. *Schizophr Res*, **29**, 160–161. Puri BK, Richardson AJ. (1998) Sustained remission of positive and negative symptoms of schizophrenia following treatment with eicosapentaenoic acid. *Arch Gen Psychiatry*, **55**, 188–189.
Try **amisulpride** (400–800mg/day) or **haloperidol** (2mg/day) or **nefazodone** (400–600mg/day)	❖ Anecdotal reports of clinical improvement. No published evidence	

Notes

✧ For discussion of augmentation strategies see Chong S-A and Remington G, (2000) Clozapine Augmentation: Safety and Efficacy. *Schizophr Bull*, **26**, 421–440.

✧ Always consider the use of mood stabilisers and/or antidepressants where mood disturbance is thought to contribute to symptoms.

Refractory schizophrenia

Alternatives to clozapine (where clozapine has proved toxic or is contra-indicated)

Treatment	Comments/references
Risperidone 4–8mg/day	Doubtful efficacy in true treatment refractory schizophrenia e.g. Breier AF, Malhotra AK, Su TP, *et al.* (1999) Clozapine and risperidone in chronic schizophrenia: effects on symptoms, Parkinsonian side effects, and neuroendocrine response. *Am J Psychiatry*, **156**, 294–298. Bondolfi G, Dufour H, Patris M, *et al.* (1998) Risperidone versus clozapine in treatment-resistant chronic schizophrenia: a randomized double-blind study. *Am J Psychiatry*, **155**, 499–504. (N.B. Treatment intolerant subjects included)
Olanzapine 5–25mg/day	Probably not effective e.g. Breier A, Hamilton SH. (1999) Comparative efficacy of olanzapine and haloperidol for patients with treatment-resistant schizophrenia. *Biol Psychiatry,* **45**, 403–411. (positive result). Conley RR, Tamminga CA, Bartko JJ, *et al.* (1998) Olanzapine compared with chlorpromazine in treatment-resistant schizophrenia. *Am J Psychiatry*, **155**, 914–920. (negative). Sanders RD, Mossman D. (1999) An open trial of olanzapine in patients with treatment-refractory psychoses. *J Clin Psychopharmacol.* **19**, 62–66. (negative). Taylor D, Mir S, Mace S. (1999) Olanzapine in practice: a prospective naturalistic study. *Psych Bull,* **23**, 178–180. (negative).
Olanzapine high dose 30–60mg/day	Possibly effective, but expensive and unlicensed. No controlled trial as yet e.g. Sheitman BB, Lindgren JC, Early J, *et al.* (1997) High-dose olanzapine for treatment-refractory schizophrenia. *Am J Psychiatry*, **154**, 1626. Fanous A, Lindenmayer JP. (1999) Schizophrenia and schizoaffective disorder treated with high doses of olanzapine. *J Clin Psychopharmacol,* **19**, 275–276. Dursun SM, Gardner DM, Bird DC, *et al.* (1999) Olanzapine for patients with treatment-resistant schizophrenia: a naturalistic case-series outcome study. *Can J Psychiatry,* **44**, 701–704. Note that olanzapine may lose atypicality at higher doses e.g. Bronson BD and Lindenmayer J-P. (2000) Adverse effects of high dose olanzapine in treatment – refractory schizophrenia. *J Clin Psychopharmacol,* **20**, 382–384 (letter).
Omega–3-triglycides	Suggested efficacy but poor data base. e.g. Mellor JE, Laugharne JDE, Peet M. (1996) Omega–3 fatty acid supplementation in schizophrenic patients. *Human Psychopharmacol,* **11**, 39–46. Puri BK, Steiner R, Richardson AJ. (1998) Sustained remission of positive and negative symptoms of schizophrenia following treatment with eicosapentaenoic acid. *Arch Gen Psychiatry*, **55**, 188–189.

Notes

✧ Judged by evidence-based criteria, only clozapine is effective in refractory schizophrenia.

✧ Above treatments should only be used instead of clozapine where clozapine cannot be used because of toxicity or very poor tolerability.

✧ Switching from clozapine to other atypicals is usually unsuccessful or disastrous and should not be attempted unless a severe clozapine-related adverse effect has occurred.

Further reading

Still DJ, Dorson PG, Crismon MH, *et al.* (1996) Effects of switching inpatients with treatment-resistant schizophrenia from clozapine to risperidone. *Psychiatric Services,* **47**, 1382–1384.
Henderson DC, Nasrallah RA, Goff DC. (1998) Switching from clozapine to olanzapine in treatment-refractory schizophrenia: safety, clinical efficacy, and predictors of response. *J Clin Psychiatry,* **59**, 585–588.

Depot medication

Advice on prescribing depot medication

✦ **Give a test dose**

Depots are long acting. Any adverse effects which result from injection are likely to be long lived. Thus a small test dose is essential to avoid severe, prolonged adverse effects. See table and manufacturer's information.

✦ **Begin with the lowest therapeutic dose**

There are few data showing clear dose-response effects for depot preparations. There is some information which indicates that low doses are at least as effective as higher ones. Low doses are likely to be better tolerated and are certainly less expensive.

✦ **Administer at the longest possible licensed interval**

All depots can be safely administered at their licensed dosing intervals. There is no evidence to suggest that shortening the dose interval improves efficacy. Moreover, injections are painful, so less frequent administration is desirable. The "observation" that some patients deteriorate in the days before the next depot is due is probably fallacious. For some hours (or even days with some preparations) plasma levels of antipsychotics continue to fall, albeit slowly, after the next injection. Thus patients are most at risk of deterioration immediately after a depot injection and not before it. Moreover, in trials, relapse seems only to occur 3-6 months after withdrawing depot therapy; roughly the time required to clear steady-state depot drug levels from the blood.

✦ **Adjust doses only after an adequate period of assessment**

Attainment of peak plasma levels, therapeutic effect and steady state plasma levels are all delayed with depot injections. Doses may be <u>reduced</u> if adverse effects occur, but should only be <u>increased</u> after careful assessment over at least one month, preferably longer. The use of adjunctive oral medication to assess depot requirements may be helpful, but it too is complicated by the slow emergence of antipsychotic effects. Note that at the start of therapy, plasma levels of antipsychotic released from a depot increase over several weeks, without increasing the given dose. Dose increases during this time to steady state plasma levels are thus illogical and impossible to evaluate properly.

Antipsychotic depot injections
Suggested doses and frequencies

Drug	Trade name	Test dose (mg)	Dose range (mg / week)	Dosing interval (weeks)	Comments
Flupenthixol decanoate	*Depixol*	20	12.5–400	2–4	? Mood elevating; may worsen agitation
Fluphenazine decanoate	*Modecate*	12.5	6.25–50	2–5	Avoid in depression High EPS
Haloperidol decanoate	*Haldol*	25*	12.5–75	4	High EPS, low incidence of sedation
Pipothiazine palmitate	*Piportil*	25	12.5–50	4	? Lower incidence of EPS (unproven)
Zuclopenthixol decanoate	*Clopixol*	100	100–600	2–4	? Useful in agitation and aggression

Notes

✧ Give a quarter or half stated doses in elderly.

✧ After test dose, wait 4–10 days before starting titration to maintenance therapy (see product information for individual drugs).

✧ Dose range is given in mg/week for convenience only – avoid using shorter dose intervals than those recommended except in exceptional circumstances, e.g.: long interval necessitates high volume (>3–4ml) injection.

✧ EPS = extrapyramidal side effects.

* Test dose not stated by manufacturer

Modified from Taylor D, Duncan D, 1995. Antipsychotic depot injections – suggested doses and frequencies. Psychiatric Bulletin; 19, 357.

Further reading

Taylor D. (1999) Depot antipsychotics revisited. *Psych Bull,* **23**, 551–553.

Clozapine – dosing regimen

Many of clozapine's adverse effects are dose-dependent and are possibly associated with a rapid increase in dose. Adverse effects also tend to be more common at the beginning of therapy. To minimise these problems it is important to start therapy at a low dose and to increase slowly.

Clozapine should be started at a dose of 12.5mg once a day. Blood pressure should be monitored hourly for six hours because of clozapine's hypotensive effect. This monitoring is not usually necessary if the first dose is given at night. On day two, the dose can be increased to 12.5mg twice daily. If the patient is tolerating the clozapine, the dose can then be increased by 25mg to 50mg a day, until a dose of 300mg a day is reached. This can usually be achieved in two to three weeks.

Further dosage increases should be made slowly in increments of 50mg to 100mg each week. A dose of 450mg/day or a plasma level of 350mcg/L should be aimed for. The total clozapine dose should be divided and, if sedation is a problem, the larger portion of the dose can be given at night.

The following table is a suggested starting regime for clozapine. This is a cautious regimen – more rapid increases have been used in exceptional circumstances. Slower titration may be necessary where sedation is severe.

Day	Morning dose (mg)	Evening dose (mg)
1	–	12.5
2	12.5	12.5
3	25	25
4	25	25
5	25	50
6	25	50
7	50	50
8	50	75
9	75	75
10	75	100
11	100	100
12	100	125
13	125	125
14	125	150
15	150	150
18	150	200
21	200	200
28	200	250

If the patient is not tolerating a particular dose, decrease to one which was being tolerated. If the adverse effect resolves, increase the dose again but at a slower rate. If for any reason a patient misses *less than* two day's clozapine, restart at the dose prescribed before the event. Do not administer extra tablets to catch up. If more than two days are missed: restart at 12.5mg once daily and increase slowly (but at a faster rate than in drug-naive patients).

Atypical antipsychotics – titration details[1]

Drug	Starting dose	Minimum effective dose	Maximum dose (may differ from manufacturer's recommendations)
Clozapine (See table)	12.5mg/day	around 300mg/day (lower in elderly)	900mg/day
Olanzapine	10mg/day (5mg in some – see product literature)	5–10mg/day	20mg/day (ceiling dose not yet defined)
Risperidone	2mg/day (1mg in elderly)	4mg/day ? lower in some (e.g. elderly)	8mg/day (higher doses should be avoided)
Quetiapine	50mg/day (25mg in elderly)	300mg/day (? lower in elderly)	750mg/day (but no evidence of improved efficacy over 300mg/day)
Amisulpride	800mg/day	800mg/day for positive symptoms. 100mg/day for negative symptoms.	1200mg/day (but no evidence of improved efficacy over 800mg)

Recommended procedure:

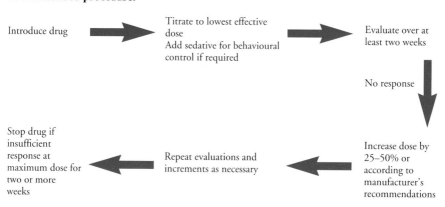

Introduce drug → Titrate to lowest effective dose. Add sedative for behavioural control if required → Evaluate over at least two weeks

No response

Increase dose by 25–50% or according to manufacturer's recommendations

Repeat evaluations and increments as necessary

Stop drug if insufficient response at maximum dose for two or more weeks

Notes

1)   Zotepine not usually considered to be atypical. Ziprasidone details not known at time of publication; not licensed in UK at time of publication.

Atypical antipsychotics – minimising costs

Atypical antipsychotics are relatively costly medicines, although their benefits may make them cost effective in practice. Cost minimisation is a practical option which reduces drug expenditure without compromising patient care or patient quality of life. It involves using the right drug for the most appropriate condition (see Protocols) and using the minimum effective dose in each patient. A guide to what is likely to be the minimum effective dose can be obtained from clinical trials using fixed doses or fixed ranges of doses of atypicals. The table below gives the cost (£/patient/30 days) in June 2000 of atypicals at their lowest effective dose, their approximate average clinical dose, and their licensed maximum dose. The table allows comparison of different doses of the same drug and of different drugs at any of the three doses. It is hoped that the table will encourage the use of lower doses of less expensive drugs, given equality in other respects and allowing for clinical need.

Atypic drugs – costs

Drug	Minimum effective dose cost [1]	Approximate clinical average dose cost [1,2]	Maximum dose cost [1]
Clozapine *N.B. No alternative available for refractory schizophrenia*	Not known – too variable	450mg/day **£241.32**	900mg/day **£482.63**
Risperidone	4mg/day **£77.22**	6mg/day **£117.00**	16mg/day **£308.88**
Olanzapine	10mg/day **£104.52**	15mg/day **£156.78**	20mg/day **£209.05**
Quetiapine	300mg/day **£113.10**	500mg/day **£169.65**	750mg/day **£254.40**
Amisulpride	400mg/day (?)[3] **£60.00**	800mg/day **£120.00**	1200mg/day **£180.00**

1) Costs are for UK adults (for 30 days) MIMS June 2000.
2) Average clinical doses are for adult inpatients in maintenance therapy.
3) Dose depends on target symptoms. Note that amisulpride is a close chemical analogue of sulpiride and shares many properties. Weak claim to atypicality.

Note also – Zotepine not usually considered to be atypical; ziprasidone details not known at time of publication; not licensed in UK at time of publication.

Equivalent doses of antipsychotics

Drug	Equivalent dose (Consensus) (mg/day)	Range of values in literature (mg/day)
Chlorpromazine	100	-
Thioridazine	100	75–100
Fluphenazine	2	2–5
Trifluoperazine	5	2.5–5
Flupenthixol	3	2–3
Zuclopenthixol	25	25–60
Haloperidol	3	1.5–5
Droperidol	4	1–4
Sulpiride	200	200–270
Pimozide	2	2
Loxapine	10	10–25
Fluphenazine *depot*	5/week	1–12.5/week
Pipothiazine *depot*	10/week	10–12.5/week
Flupenthixol *depot*	10/week	10–20/week
Zuclopenthixol *depot*	100/week	40–100/week
Haloperidol *depot*	15/week	5–25/week

Note – all values should be regarded as approximate
Dose equivalencies are not relevant to atypical drugs: therapeutic doses are well defined.

Antipsychotics – maximum doses

Drug	Maximum dose (mg/day)
Chlorpromazine	1000
Thioridazine	800 (see BNF)
Fluphenazine	20
Trifluoperazine	None (suggest 50)
Flupenthixol	18
Zuclopenthixol	150
Haloperidol	120
Droperidol	120
Sulpiride	2400
Pimozide	20
Loxapine	250
Clozapine	900
Risperidone	16
Amisulpride	1200
Olanzapine	20
Zotepine	300
Ziprasidone	160?
Quetiapine	750
Fluphenazine *depot*	50/week
Pipothiazine *depot*	50/week
Haloperidol *depot*	300 every 4 weeks
Flupenthixol *depot*	400/week
Zuclopenthixol *depot*	600/week

Note

Doses above these maxima should only be used in extreme circumstances: there is no evidence for improved efficacy. Always follow RCP guidelines.

Oral/parenteral dose equivalents

Drug	Oral dose (mg)	Equivalent IM or IV dose (mg)
Antipsychotics		
Chlorpromazine	100	25–50*
Droperidol	10	7.5
Haloperidol	10	5
Promazine	100	100
Anticholinergics		
Procyclidine	10	7.5

* IM/IV chlorpromazine not recommended

Note

Because of the variation in bioavailability with some drugs, prescriptions should always specify the dose and a single route of administration.

For example:

Droperidol 10mg IM Q6H PRN

III

Treatment of
Affective Illness

Antidepressant drugs

Tricyclic	Main indication	Alternative indications (#not licensed)	Dosing	Adverse effects/ contraindications
Amitriptyline	Depression	Enuresis in children Migraine prophylaxis# Anxiolytic#	25–150mg/day (once daily) child > 7 yrs 10-20mg daily	Sedation, often with hangover; postural hypotension; tachycardia/ arrhythmias; dry mouth, blurred vision, constipation, retention C/I: prostatism, narrow angle glaucoma, post MI, heart block. Caution in epilepsy, liver disease
Nortriptyline	Depression	As for amitriptyline	20–150mg once daily	As for amitriptyline, but less sedative, less anticholinergic, no postural hypotension
Dothiepin	Depression	None	75–225mg once daily	As for amitriptyline
Imipramine	Depression	As for amitriptyline	75–200mg 300mg max in inpatients once daily	As for amitriptyline, but less sedative
Desipramine	Depression	None	75–200mg once daily	As for nortriptyline, hypotension may occur
Clomipramine	Depression	Obsessive comp-ulsive disorder Phobic states Cataplexy associated with narcolepsy	10–250mg once daily	As for amitriptyline
Lofepramine	Depression	None	70–210mg/day BD or TDS	As amitriptyline, but less sedative/anticholinergic/ cardiotoxic
Trimipramine	Depression – including that associated with anxiety	None	75–300mg once daily	As for amitriptyline, but more sedative

Interactions	Half life (hrs)	Cost (£)	Comments
Alcohol Anticholinergics (inc neuroleptics, etc) MAOIs Sympathomimetics Cimetidine	8–24	0.04/50mg	Due to long $t_{1/2}$,SR preparations unnecessary Metabolised to nortriptyline Liquid form available
As for amitriptyline	18–96	0.11/25mg	Good **mildly** sedating antidepressant; particularly useful in the elderly
As for amitriptyline	11–40	0.15/75mg	Very similar to amitriptyline: structure only differs by replacing C with S atom in tricyclic ring. Very dangerous in overdose. Liquid form available
As for amitriptyline	4–18	0.04/25mg	Metabolised to desipramine. Liquid form available
As for amitriptyline	12–24	0.04/25mg.	Not currently marketed in UK but widely used elsewhere
As for amitriptyline	17–28	0.12/50mg	Liquid form available
As for amitriptyline	1.5–6	0.18/70mg	Metabolised to desipramine. **Safer in overdose** Liquid available
As for amitriptyline Safer with MAOIs than other tricyclics	7–23	0.30/50mg	Most sedating antidepressant

Antidepressant drugs

SSRIs	Main indication	Alternative indications (#not licensed)	Dosing	Adverse effects/ contraindications
Fluvoxamine	Depression	OCD	100–300mg/day BD if > 100mg	Nausea, diarrhoea, agitation, insomnia, dry mouth & blurred vision, tremor, dizziness, hyponatraemia, sexual dysfunction (male and female). Somnolence may occur rarely Caution in epilepsy
Fluoxetine	Depression – including that associated with anxiety	Bulimia, OCD, Premenstrual dysphoric disorder	20mg /day (depression) 60mg /day (bulimia) 20–60mg/day (OCD)	As fluvoxamine, but: weight loss and rash may occur. Insomnia and agitation possibly more common. Hypoglycaemia may occur rarely: avoid in diabetes. Vasculitis may occur very rarely
Sertraline	Depression – including that associated with anxiety	Preventing relapse of depressive illness, OCD	50–100mg once daily 150–200mg/day may be used	As fluvoxamine, but nausea less common. Contra-indicated in hepatic failure, caution in renal failure
Paroxetine	Depression – including that associated with anxiety	OCD Panic Disorder +/- agoraphobia Social phobia	20–50mg/day (depression) 20–60mg/day (OCD) 10–50mg/day (panic disorder)	As fluvoxamine, but: sedation more likely. Extra-pyramidal symptoms more common, but rare. Withdrawal effects common
Citalopram	Depression	Preventing relapse of depressive illness Panic disorder +/- agoraphobia	20–60mg once daily	As fluvoxamine, but: nausea may be less common

Interactions	Half-life (hrs)	Cost (£)	Comments
Inhibits hepatic demethylation: (CYP1A2). Caution with TCAs, warfarin, phenytoin, clozapine theophylline; MAOIs never. Care with lithium, tryptophan, alcohol	15 single dose 17–22 multiple dose	0.63/100mg	Safe in overdose (this applies to all SSRIs). Relatively high incidence of nausea reported in some trials and observed in clinical practice
As fluvoxamine but safe with theophylline. Inhibits CYP2D6, CYP3A4. MAOIs / tryptophan never. Increases plasma levels of tricyclics, benzos, clozapine and cyclosporin. No interaction with alcohol	24–140	0.37/20mg (generic)	Undoubted efficacy but not useful where degree of sedation is required. Active metabolite has $t_{1/2}$ of 7–9 days. Wide range of interactions reported. Liquid form available
As fluvoxamine but safe with theophylline. Inhibits CYP2D6. Care with lithium/ tryptophan, alcohol. MAOIs never. Alcohol – caution	24–26	0.95/100mg (0.58/50 mg)	Less potent inhibitor of CYP2D6 but some interactions reported
As fluoxetine. Safe with theophylline and alcohol. Inhibits CYP2D6. MAOIs never	24	0.59/20mg	No active metabolites Withdrawal reaction more frequently reported – withdraw very slowly Liquid form available
Few interactions reported. MAOIs never. Safe with alcohol	33	0.57/20mg	Poor inhibitor of CYP2D6 and so may cause fewer adverse drug interactions

MAOIs	Main indication	Alternative indications (#not licensed)	Dosing	Adverse effects/ contraindications
Phenelzine	Depression	Anxiety states# Obsessive compulsive disorder#	15–30mg tds	Anticholinergic effects Nervousness Weight gain, hypotension Hepatotoxicity, oedema Leucopenia Psychosis CI: CVS disease, Phaeochromocytoma Liver disease Diabetes
Tranyl-cypromine	Depression	As for phenelzine	10mg b.d. Max. 30mg/day BD total dose before mid pm	As for phenelzine but even more caution required Additionally, hyperthyroidism, insomnia Hepatotoxicity and weight gain less common
Isocarboxazid	Depression	As for phenelzine	30–60mg loading for six weeks 10–20mg maintenance once daily	As for phenelzine but may cause weight loss, more hepatotoxicity, less hypotension
Moclobemide	Major depressive illness	Social phobia	300–600mg/day BD after food Last dose before 3.00pm	Insomnia, nausea, agitation, confusion Hypertension reported – may be related to tyramine ingestion

Interactions	Half life (hrs)	Cost (£)	Comments
Tyramine in food Always carry an MAOI card Sympathomimetics Opioids Tricyclics Tryptophan SSRIs Venlafaxine	1.5	0.20/15mg	Phenelzine is possibly the safest of MAOI's and is the one that should be used if combinations are being considered
As for phenelzine, only more severe and never with tricyclics	2.5	0.05/10mg	Mild dependence, amphetamine-like structure ? metabolised to amphetamine. More potent adverse effects, never use in combination
As for phenelzine	36	0.49/10mg	Similar to phenelzine except longer half life
Tyramine interactions rare and mild Opioid interactions limited to pethidine and ? codeine Avoid: sympathomimetics, SSRIs, clomipramine, l-dopa Caution: TCAs, lithium, sumatriptan Cimetidine – use half dose of moclobemide	1–2	0.33/150mg	Reversible inhibitor of MAOI-A. Fewer adverse effects, fewer drug interactions. Food interactions possible if high doses (>600mg/day) used or if large quantities of tyramine ingested

Antidepressant drugs

Drug	Main indication	Alternative indications	Dosing	Adverse effects / contraindications
Trazodone	Depression – including that associated with anxiety	None	150–600mg/day once daily (bd above 300mg)	As amitriptyline, but not anticholinergic, less cardiotoxic
Nefazodone	Depression – including that associated with anxiety	None	200–600mg/day (BD)	As trazodone, but less sedative, less hypotensive
Venlafaxine	Depressive illness	None	75–375mg daily (BD) after food XL prep is OD, max dose 225mg/day	Nausea, insomnia, dry mouth, sexual dysfunction, drowsiness, headache. Elevation of blood pressure at higher doses. Discontinue if rash occurs. Halve dose in hepatic/renal impairment. Withdrawal effects are common even if doses are a few hours late
Reboxetine	Treatment of depression and maintenance of improvement	None, but limited data to suggest reboxetine improves social functioning	8–12mg/day (BD)	Insomnia, sweating, dizziness, dry mouth, constipation, urinary hesitation
Mirtazapine	Depression	None	15–45mg/day As single dose at night	Drowsiness (low dose), increased appetite, weight gain. Rarely, blood dyscrasias, LFT changes, convulsions, myoclonus, oedema

Interactions	Half life (hrs)	Cost	Comments
As amitriptyline but safer in epilepsy	1–13	0.36/100mg	Sedative, not anticholinergic Priapism possible Liquid available
Potent inhibitor of CYP3A4. See Data Sheet	2–4	0.30/200mg	Sexual dysfunction rarely reported
Few reported Care with lithium MAOIs – never Care with cimetidine Minor effect on CYP enzymes	5 (11 for active metabolite)	0.86/75mg	Limited data to support special properties of venlafaxine: fast onset; greater efficacy; efficacy in refractory illness Further studies/clinical experiences needed to confirm or refute these See section on refractory depression
Information is incomplete Minor effect on CYP2D6/3A4 MAOIs – never No interaction with alcohol	13	0.32/4mg tab	Impotence is rare, occurs mainly in men and is dose-related Safe in overdose
Minimal effect on CYP2D6/1A2/3A Avoid with other sedatives including alcohol MAOIs – never	20–40	0.82/30mg tab	Appears safe in overdose, sexual dysfunction is rare

Depression in primary care – golden rules of prescribing

1. **Discuss with patient choice of drug and, when necessary, other therapies**. (See CAAT system in Appendix 2.)

2. **Prescribe a recognised effective dose of antidepressant** (after careful titration where necessary). (See page 60 for recommended doses.)

3. **Continue treatment for at least 4–6 months after resolution of symptoms**.

4. **Withdraw gradually** over 2–4 weeks, or longer if necessary.

Drug treatment of depression

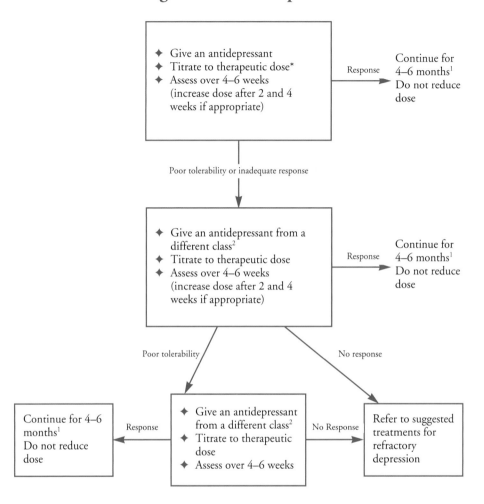

Give an antidepressant
- ✦ Give an antidepressant
- ✦ Titrate to therapeutic dose*
- ✦ Assess over 4–6 weeks
  (increase dose after 2 and 4
  weeks if appropriate)

Response → Continue for 4–6 months[1]
Do not reduce dose

Poor tolerability or inadequate response

- ✦ Give an antidepressant from a
  different class[2]
- ✦ Titrate to therapeutic dose
- ✦ Assess over 4–6 weeks
  (increase dose after 2 and 4
  weeks if appropriate)

Response → Continue for 4–6 months[1]
Do not reduce dose

Poor tolerability   *No response*

- ✦ Give an antidepressant
  from a different class[2]
- ✦ Titrate to therapeutic
  dose
- ✦ Assess over 4–6 weeks

Response → Continue for 4–6 months[1]
Do not reduce dose

No Response → Refer to suggested treatments for refractory depression

Notes

＊   Established *minimum* therapeutic doses as follows:

Lofepramine	140mg/day
Tricyclics	125mg/day
Citalopram	20mg/day
Fluoxetine	20mg/day
Fluvoxamine	100mg/day
Paroxetine	20mg/day
Sertraline	50mg/day
Mirtazapine	30mg/day
Moclobemide	300mg/day
Reboxetine	8mg/day
Venlafaxine	75mg/day

Note: Higher doses may be required. See table on pages 50–58 or BNF.

1.   After 1st episode, continue for 4–6 months after symptom resolution. For subsequent episodes consider longer treatment periods.

> See: American Psychiatric Association. (1993) Practice guideline for major depressive disorder in adults. *Am J Psychiatry*, **150**, 1–26.
> Crismon ML, Trivedi M, Pigott TA, *et al.* (1999) The Texas medication algorithm project: report of the Texas Consensus Conference panel on medication treatment of major depressive disorder.
> Anderson IM, Nutt DJ, Deakin JFW. (2000) Evidence-based guidelines for treating depressive disorders with antidepressants: a revision of the 1993 British Association for Psychopharmacology guidelines. *J Psychopharmacol*, **14**, 3–20.

2.   Switching <u>between</u> classes has a theoretical and clinical basis in non-response and is especially appropriate where previous drugs were poorly tolerated. Switching <u>within</u> classes may also be effective in non-responders.

> See: Nelson JC. (1998) Treatment of antidepressant nonresponders: Augmentation or switch? (1998) *J Clin Psychiatry*, **59** (suppl 15), 35–41.
> Joffe RT. (1999) Substitution therapy in patients with major depression. *CNS Drugs*, **11**, 175–180.

Suggestions for treatment of refractory depression

1st choice – Commonly used treatments generally well-supported by published literature

Treatment	Advantages	Disadvantages	References
Add **lithium** Aim for plasma level of 0.4–0.6mmol/L	❖ Well established ❖ Effective in around half of cases ❖ Well supported in the literature	❖ Sometimes poorly tolerated at higher plasma levels ❖ Potentially toxic ❖ Usually needs specialist referral ❖ Plasma monitoring is essential	See Fava M, Rosenbaum JF, McGrath PJ, *et al.* (1994) Lithium and tricyclic augmentation of fluoxetine treatment. *Am J Psychiatry*, **151**, 1372–1374 Dinan TG. (1993) Lithium augmentation in sertraline-resistant depression: a preliminary dose-response study. *Acta Psychiatr Scand* **88**, 300–301 **For review see:** Bauer M, Döpfmer S. (1999) Lithium augmentation in treatment-resistant depression: meta-analysis of placebo-controlled studies. *J Clin Psychopharmacol*, **19**, 427–434
Electroconvulsive therapy	❖ Well established ❖ Effective ❖ Well supported in the literature	❖ Poor reputation in public domain ❖ Necessitates general anaesthetic ❖ Needs specialist referral	See Folkerts HW, Michael N, Tölle R, *et al.* (1997) Electroconvulsive therapy vs paroxetine in treatment-resistant depression – a randomized study. *Acta Psychiatr Scand*, **96**, 334–342
Venlafaxine (high dose) (> 200mg/day)	❖ Usually well tolerated ❖ Can be initiated in primary care	❖ Limited support in literature ❖ Nausea and vomiting ❖ Discontinuation reactions common ❖ Blood pressure monitoring essential	Poiriere MF, Boyer P. (1999) Venlafaxine and paroxetine in treatment-resistant depression. *Br J Psychiatry*, **175**, 12–16 Nierenberg AA, Feighner JP, Rudolph R, *et al.* (1994) Venlafaxine for treatment-resistant unipolar depression. *J Clin Psychopharmacol*, **14**, 419–423
Add **tri-iodothyronine** (20–50µg/day)	❖ Usually well tolerated ❖ Moderate literature support	❖ TFT monitoring required ❖ Usually needs specialist referral	See Joffe RT, Singer W. (1990) A comparison of tri-iodothyronine and thyroxine in the potentiation of tricyclic antidepressants. *Psychiatry Research*, **32**, 241–251
Add **tryptophan** 2–3g tds	❖ Usually well tolerated ❖ Well researched	❖ Danger of serotonin syndrome ❖ Theoretical risk of Eosinophilia-myalgia syndrome ❖ Patient and prescriber must register with manufacturers ❖ Data relate mainly to combination with tricyclics/MAOIs	Smith S. (1998) Tryptophan in the treatment of resistant depression – a review. *Pharm Journal*, 261, 819–821

Suggestions for treatment of refractory depression – *continued*

2nd choice – Less commonly used, variably supported by published evaluations

Treatment	Advantages	Disadvantages	References
Add **pindolol** (5mg tds)	❖ Well tolerated ❖ Well researched ❖ Can be initiated in primary care	❖ Literature somewhat contradictory ❖ Data relate mainly to acceleration of response (evidence is more compelling)	McAskill R, Mir S, Taylor D. (1998) Pindolol augmentation of antidepressant therapy. *B J Psychiatry*, **173**, 203–208. Räsänen P, Hakko H, Tuhonen J. (1999) Pindolol and major affective disorders: a three-year follow-up study of 30,483 patients. *J Clin Psychopharmacol*, **19**, 297–302
Add **dexamethasone** (4mg daily for 4/7)	❖ Well tolerated ❖ Short course	❖ Little clinical experience ❖ Very limited literature support	Dinan TG, Lavelle E, Cooney J, *et al.* (1997) Dexamethasone augmentation in treatment-resistant depression *Acta Psychiatr Scand*, **95**, 58–61. Bodani M, Sheehan B, Philpot M. (1999) the use of dexamethasone in elderly patients with antidepressant-resistant depressive illness. *J Psychopharmacol*, 13: 196–197
Add or try **lamotrigine** (aim for 200mg/day but lower doses may be effective)	❖ Probably effective	❖ Risk of rash ❖ Slow titration ❖ Sparse literature	Calabrese JR, Bowden CL, Sachs GS. (1999) A double-blind placebo-controlled study of lamotrigine monotherapy in outpatients with bipolar I depression. *J Clin Psychiatry* **60**: 79–88. Maltese TM. (1999) Adjunctive lamotrigine treatment for major depression. *Am J Psychiatry*, **156**, 1833 (letter).
❖ **High dose tricyclics** e.g. imipramine 300mg/day	❖ Widely used (especially in USA) ❖ Inexpensive	❖ Danger of ECG abnormalities ❖ ECG monitoring essential	Malhi GS, Bridges PK. (1997) Management of resistant depression. *Int J Psychiatry in Clin Practice*, **1**, 269–276.
❖ **MAOI + TCA** e.g. Trimipramine + phenelzine	❖ Widely used in 1960s, and 1970s ❖ Inexpensive	❖ Potential for dangerous interaction ❖ Becoming less popular	White K, Simpson G. (1984) The combined use of MAOIs and tricyclics. *J Clin Psychiatry*, **45**, 67–69.

Other reported treatments – may be worth trying, but limited published support

❖ Add bupropion 300mg/day	Fatemi SH, Emamian ES, Kist DA. (1999) Venlafaxine and bupropion combination therapy in a case of treatment-resistant depression. *Ann Pharmacother*, **33**, 701–703. Pierre JM, Gitlin MJ. (2000) Buproprion-tranylcypromine combination for treatment – refractory depression. *J Clin Psych*, **61**, 449–450.
❖ Add buspirone 30mg/day	Fischer P, Tauscher J, Küfferle, *et al.* (1998) Weak antidepressant response after buspirone augmentation of serotonin reuptake inhibitors in refractory severe depression. *Int Clin Psychopharmacol.* **13**, 83–86.
❖ Add clonazepam 0.5–1.0mg at night	Smith WT, Londborg PD, Glaudin V, *et al.* (1998) Short-term augmentation of fluoxetine with clonazepam in the treatment of depression: a double-blind study. *Am J Psychiatry*, **155**, 1339–1345.
❖ Add mirtazapine 15–30mg ON	Carpenter LL, Jocic Z, Hall JM, *et al.* (1999) Mirtazapine augmentation in the treatment of refractory depression. *J Clin Psychiatry*, **60**, 45–49.
❖ Add modafinil 100–200mg/day	Menza MA, Kaufman KR, Castellanos A. (2000) Modafinil augmentation of antidepressant treatment in depression. *J Clin Psychiatry*, **61**, 378–381.
❖ Add olanzapine 10–15mg/day	Weisler RH, Ahearn EP, Davidson JRT, *et al.* (1997) Adjunctive use of olanzapine in mood disorders: five case reports. *Annals of Clin Psychiatry*, **9**, 259–261.
❖ Add risperidone 0.5–1.0mg/day	Ostroff RB, Nelson JC. (1999) Risperidone augmentation of selective serotonin reuptake inhibitors in major depression. *J Clin Psychiatry*, **60**, 256–259. Stoll AL, Haura G. (2000) Tranylcypromine plus risperidone for treatment refractory major depression. *J Clin Psychopharmacol*, **20**, 495–497 (letter).
❖ Ketoconazole 400–800mg/day	Wolkowitz OM, Reus VI, Chan T, *et al.* (1999) Antiglucocorticoid treatment of depression: double-blind ketoconazole. *Biol Psychiatry*, **45**, 1070–1074.
❖ Oestrogens (various regimes used)	Stahl SM. (1998) Basic psychopharmacology of antidepressants, Part 2: oestrogen as an adjunct to antidepressant treatment. *J Clin Psychiatry*, **59** (suppl 4), 15–24.
❖ SSRI + TCA e.g. citalopram 20mg/day with amitriptyline 50mg/day	Taylor D. (1995) Selective serotonin reuptake inhibitors and tricyclic antidepressants in combination: interactions and therapeutic uses. *Br J Psychiatry*, **167**, 575–580.

Antidepressants – swapping and stopping

General guidelines

1. All antidepressants have the potential to cause withdrawal phenomena. When taken continuously *for six weeks or longer,* antidepressants should not be stopped abruptly unless a serious adverse effect has occurred (e.g. cardiac arrhythmia with a tricyclic).

2. Antidepressants should be withdrawn slowly, preferably over four weeks, by weekly decrements. Note that some patients will prefer abrupt withdrawal, preferring to avoid suffering prolonged, if mild, discontinuation reactions.

Examples:		Decrements			
Drug	**Maintenance dose** (mg/day)	**Dose after 1ˢᵗ** (mg/day)	**Dose after 2ⁿᵈ** (mg/day)	**Dose after 3ʳᵈ** (mg/day)	**Dose after 4ᵗʰ** (mg/day)
Amitriptyline	150	100	50	25	Nil
Paroxetine	30	20	10	5 mg (liquid)	Nil
Trazodone	450	300	150	75	Nil

3. Fluoxetine, because of its long plasma half-life and active metabolite, may be stopped abruptly if the dose is 20mg/day.

4. If withdrawal symptoms occur (see below) slow the rate of drug withdrawal or (if drug has been stopped) give reassurance: symptoms rarely last more than 1–2 weeks. Restarting is only recommended if withdrawal is severe or prolonged.

Antidepressant discontinuation syndrome

Symptoms

Dizziness*

Electric shock sensations*

Anxiety and agitation

Insomnia

Flu-like symptoms

Diarrhoea and abdominal spasms

Paraesthesia*

Mood swings

Nausea

Low mood

* Common in SSRI/venlafaxine withdrawal

---

5.   When swapping from one antidepressant to another, abrupt withdrawal should usually be avoided. Cross-tapering is preferred, where the dose of the ineffective or poorly tolerated drug is slowly reduced while the new drug is slowly introduced.

Example:		Week 1	Week 2	Week 3	Week 4
Withdrawing Dothiepin	150mg OD	100mg OD	50mg OD	25mg OD	Nil
Introducing Citalopram	Nil	10mg OD	10mg OD	20mg OD	20mg OD

✦   The speed of cross-tapering is best judged by monitoring patient tolerability. No clear guidelines are available, so caution is required.

✦   Note that the co-administration of some antidepressants, even when cross-tapering, is absolutely contra-indicated. In other cases, theoretical risks or lack of experience preclude recommending cross-tapering.

✦   In some cases cross-tapering may not be considered necessary. An example is when switching from one SSRI to another: their effects are so similar that administration of the second drug is likely to ameliorate withdrawal effects of the first. However, there is little firm evidence of this occurring.

✦   Potential dangers of simultaneously administering two antidepressants include pharmacodynamic interactions (serotonin syndrome, hypotension, drowsiness) and pharmacokinetic interactions (e.g. elevation of tricyclic plasma levels by some SSRIs). See below for symptoms of serotonin syndrome.

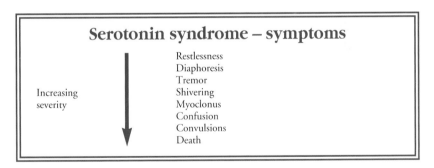

See: Mir S & Taylor D. (1999) Serotonin Syndrome *Psych Bull*, **23**, 742–747.

From \ To	MAOIs – hydrazines	Tranyl-cypromine	Tricyclics	Citalopram	Fluoxetine	Paroxetine
MAOIs – hydrazines	Withdraw and wait for two weeks	Withdraw and wait for two weeks	Withdraw and wait for two weeks	Withdraw and wait for two weeks	Withdraw and wait for two weeks	Withdraw and wait for two weeks
Tranyl-cypromine	Withdraw and wait for two weeks	–	Withdraw and wait for two weeks	Withdraw and wait for two weeks	Withdraw and wait for two weeks	Withdraw and wait for two weeks
Tricyclics	Withdraw and wait for one week	Withdraw and wait for one week	Cross taper cautiously	Halve dose and add citalopram then slow withdrawal[*2]	Halve dose and add fluoxetine then slow withdrawal[*2]	Halve dose and add paroxetine then slow withdrawal[*2]
Citalopram	Withdraw and wait for one week	Withdraw and wait for one week	Cross taper cautiously [*2]	–	Withdraw then start fluoxetine	Withdraw and start paroxetine at 10mg/day
Paroxetine	Withdraw and wait for two weeks	Withdraw and wait for one week	Cross taper cautiously with very low dose of tricyclic [*2]	Withdraw and start citalopram	Withdraw then start fluoxetine	–
Fluoxetine[*3]	Withdraw and wait five to six weeks	Withdraw and wait five to six weeks	Stop fluoxetine. Start tricyclic at very low dose and increase very slowly	Stop fluoxetine Wait 4–7 days Start citalopram at 10mg/day and increase slowly	–	Stop fluoxetine Wait 4–7 days, then start paroxetine 10mg/day

Sertraline	Trazodone/ nefazodone	Moclobemide	Reboxetine	Venlafaxine	Mirtazapine
Withdraw and wait for two weeks	Withdraw and wait for two weeks	Withdraw and wait for two weeks[*1]	Withdraw and wait for two weeks	Withdraw and wait for two weeks	Withdraw and wait for two weeks
Withdraw and wait for two weeks	Withdraw and wait for two weeks	Withdraw and wait for two weeks[*1]	Withdraw and wait for two weeks	Withdraw and wait for two weeks	Withdraw and wait for two weeks
Halve dose and add sertraline then slow withdrawal[*2]	Halve dose and add trazodone/ nefazodone, then slow withdrawal	Withdraw and wait for one week	Cross taper cautiously	Cross taper cautiously, starting with venlafaxine 37.5mg/day	Withdraw before starting mirtazapine cautiously
Withdraw and start sertraline at 25mg/day	Withdraw before starting titration of trazodone/ nefazodone	Withdraw and wait at least one week	Cross taper cautiously	Withdraw Start venlafaxine 37.5mg/day Increase very slowly	Withdraw before starting mirtazapine cautiously
Withdraw and start sertraline at 25mg/day	Withdraw before starting titration of trazodone/ nefazodone	Withdraw and wait at least two weeks	Cross taper cautiously	Withdraw paroxetine Start venlafaxine 37.5mg/day and increase very slowly	Withdraw before starting mirtazapine cautiously
Stop fluoxetine Wait 4–7 days, then start sertraline 25mg/day	Stop fluoxetine Wait 4–7 days then start low dose trazodone/ nefazodone	Withdraw and wait at least five weeks	Withdraw Start reboxetine at 2mg bd and increase cautiously	Withdraw Wait 4–7 days Start venlafaxine at 37.5mg/ day Increase very slowly	Withdraw Wait 4–7 days before starting mirtazapine cautiously

Antidepressants

From \ To	MAOIs – hydrazines	Tranyl-cypromine	Tricyclics	Citalopram	Fluoxetine	Paroxetine
Sertraline	Withdraw and wait for two weeks[1]	Withdraw and wait for two weeks	Cross taper cautiously with very low dose of tricyclic[2]	Withdraw then start citalopram	Withdraw then start fluoxetine	Withdraw then start paroxetine
Trazodone/ nefazodone	Withdraw and wait at least one week	Withdraw and wait at least one week	Cross taper cautiously with very low dose of tricyclic	Withdraw then start citalopram	Withdraw then start fluoxetine	Withdraw then start paroxetine
Moclobemide	Withdraw and wait 24 hours	Withdraw and wait 24 hours	Withdraw and wait 24 hours	Withdraw and wait 24 hours	Withdraw and wait 24 hours	Withdraw and wait 24 hours
Reboxetine	Withdraw and wait at least one week	Withdraw and wait at least one week	Cross taper cautiously	Cross taper cautiously	Cross taper cautiously	Cross taper cautiously
Venlafaxine	Withdraw and wait at least one week	Withdraw and wait at least one week	Cross taper cautiously with very low dose of tricyclic[2]	Cross taper cautiously Start with 10mg/day	Cross taper cautiously Start with 20mg every other day	Cross taper cautiously Start with 10mg/day
Mirtazapine	Withdraw and wait for one week	Withdraw and wait for one week	Withdraw then start tricyclic	Withdraw then start citalopram	Withdraw then start fluoxetine	Withdraw then start paroxetine
Stopping[4]	Reduce over four weeks	Reduce over four weeks	Reduce over four weeks	Reduce over four weeks	At 20mg/day – just stop At 40mg/day reduce over two weeks	Reduce over four weeks or longer, if necessary[5]

*1. Abrupt switching is possible but not recommended.
*2. Do not co-administer clomipramine and SSRIs or venlafaxine. Withdraw clomipramine before starting.
*3. Beware interactions with fluoxetine may still occur for five weeks after stopping fluoxetine because of long half-life.

– swapping and stopping *(Continued)*

Sertraline	Trazodone/nefazodone	Moclobemide	Reboxetine	Venlafaxine	Mirtazapine˜
–	Withdraw before starting trazodone/nefazodone	Withdraw and wait at least two weeks	Cross taper cautiously	Withdraw. Start venlafaxine at 37.5mg/day	Withdraw before starting mirtazapine cautiously
Withdraw then start sertraline	–	Withdraw and wait at least one week	Withdraw, start reboxetine at 2mg BD and increase cautiously	Withdraw. Start venlafaxine at 37.5mg/day	Withdraw before starting mirtazapine cautiously
Withdraw and wait 24 hours	Withdraw and wait 24 hours	–	Withdraw and wait 24 hours	Withdraw and wait 24 hours	Withdraw and wait 24 hours
Cross taper cautiously	Cross taper cautiously	Withdraw and wait at least one week	–	Cross taper cautiously	Cross taper cautiously
Cross taper cautiously Start with 25mg/day	Cross taper cautiously	Withdraw and wait at least one week	Cross taper cautiously	–	Withdraw before starting mirtazapine cautiously
Withdraw then start sertraline	Withdraw then start trazodone/nefazodone	Withdraw and wait one week	Withdraw then start reboxetine	Withdraw then start venlafaxine	–
Reduce over four weeks	Reduce over four weeks	Reduce over four weeks	Reduce over four weeks	Reduce over four weeks or longer, if necessary*5	Reduce over four weeks

*4. See general guidelines.
*5. Withdrawal effects seem to be more pronounced. Slow withdrawal over 1-3 months may be necessary.

Cardiac effects

Drug	Heart rate	Blood pressure	QTc
Tricyclics[1]	Increase in heart rate	Low doses ↑ bp, higher doses – postural hypotension	Prolongation of QTc interval
Lofepramine[1,2]	Modest ↑ in heart rate	Less ↓ in postural bp compared with other TCAs	Can possibly ↑ QTc interval at higher doses. *(desipramine is main metabolite)*
MAOIs[1]	Decrease in heart rate	Postural hypotension Risk of hypertensive crisis	Can shorten QTc interval
Fluoxetine[3,4,5]	Small ↓ in mean heart rate	Minimal effect on bp	No effect on QTc interval
Paroxetine[6,7]	Small ↓ in mean heart rate	Minimal effect on bp	No effect on QTc interval
Sertraline[8]	Minimal effect on heart rate	Minimal effect on bp	No effect on QTc interval
Citalopram[9]	Small ↓ in heart rate	Slight ↓ in systolic bp	No effect on QTc interval
Fluvoxamine[10]	Minimal effect on heart rate	Small drops in systolic bp	No significant effect on QTc interval
Venlafaxine[11]	Marginally increased	Some postural ↓ bp. At higher doses ↑ in bp	Possible prolongation in overdose
Mirtazapine[12]	Minimal change in heart rate	Minimal effect on bp	No effect on QTc interval
Reboxetine[13,14]	Significant ↑ in heart rate	Marginal ↑ in both systolic and diastolic bp. Postural ↓ at higher doses	Unclear
Moclobemide[15,16]	Marginal ↓ in heart rate	Minimal effect on bp. Isolated cases of hypertensive episodes	No effect on QTc interval
Nefazodone[17]	Small ↓ in heart rate	Reports of postural hypotension	No effect on QTc interval
Trazodone[1]	↓ in heart rate more common although ↑ can also occur	Can cause significant postural hypotension	Can prolong QTc interval

References

1. Warrington SJ, Padgham C, Lader M. (1989) The cardiovascular effects of antidepressants. *Psychol Med*, Monograph Supplement 16, Cambridge University Press.
2. Stern H, Konetschny J, Herrmann L, *et al.* (1985) Cardiovascular effects of single doses of the antidepressants amitriptyline and lofepramine in healthy subjects. *Pharmacopsychiatry*, **18**, 272–277.
3. Fisch C. (1985) Effect of Fluoxetine on the Electrocardiogram. *J Clin Psychiatry*, **46**, 42–44.
4. Ellison ME, Milofsky JE, Ely E. (1990) Fluoxetine-induced bradycardia and syncope in two patients. *J Clin Psychiatry*, **51**, 385–386.
5. Roose SP, Glassman AH, Attia E, *et al.* (1998) Cardiovascular effects of Fluoxetine in depressed patients with heart disease. *Am J Psychiatry*, **155**, 660–665.
6. Kuhs H, Rudolf GA. (1990) Cardiovascular effects of paroxetine. *Psychopharmacology*, **102**, 379–382.
7. Roose SP, Laghrissi-Thode F, Kennedy JS, *et al.* (1998) Comparison of paroxetine and nortriptyline in depressed patients with ischemic heart disease. *JAMA*, **279**, 287–291.
8. Shapiro PA, Lespérance F, Frasure-Smith N, *et al.* (1999) An open-label preliminary trial of sertraline for treatment of major depression after acute myocardial infarction (the SADHAT trial). *Am Heart J*, **137**, 1100–1106.

# of antidepressants

Arrhythmias	Conduction disturbance	Licensed restrictions post MI	Comments
Class I anti-arrhythmic activity	Slows down cardiac conduction	CI in patients with recent MI	TCAs affect cardiac contractility. Association with sudden death
May occur at higher doses	Benign effect on cardiac conduction	CI in patients with recent MI	Less cardiotoxic than other TCAs. Reasons unclear
May cause arrhythmias and ↓ LVF	No clear effect on cardiac conduction	Use with caution in patients with cardiovascular disease	
Few cases reported in literature	None	Caution.Clinical experience is limited	
None	None	General caution in cardiac patients	
None	None	None	Only antidepressant studied in patients with recent MI
None	None	Caution, although no ECG changes	Minor metabolite which may ↑ QTc interval
None	None	Caution	Limited changes in ECG have been observed
Some reports of cardiac arrhythmias	Rare reports of conduction abnormalities	Caution. Has not been evaluated in post MI patients	
None	None	Caution in patients with recent MI	
Rhythm abnormalities may occur	Atrial and ventricular ectopic beats, especially in the elderly	Caution in patients with cardiac disease	
None	None	None	
Asymptomatic sinus bradycardia occasionally reported	Does not appear to alter cardiac conduction.	Caution in patients with recent MI	
Several case reports of arrhythmias	May have a minimal effect on cardiac conduction	Care in patients with severe cardiac disease	May be arrhythmogenic in patients with pre-existing cardiac disease

9. Rasmussen SL, Overø KF, Tanghøj P. (1999) Cardiac safety of citalopram: Prospective trials and retrospective analyses. *J Clin Psychopharmacol,* **19**, 407–415.
10. Strik JJ, Honig A, Lousberg R, *et al.* (1998) Cardiac side effects of two selective serotonin reuptake inhibitors in middle-aged and elderly patients. *Int Clin Psychopharmacol,* **13**, 263–267.
11. ABPI. (1999) Venlafaxine SPC. *Compendium of Data Sheets and Summaries of Product Characteristics.*
12. Montgomery SA. (1995) Safety of mirtazapine: a review. *Int Clin Psychopharmacol,* **10**, suppl 4, 37–45.
13. Mucci M .(1997) Reboxetine: a review of antidepressant tolerability. *J Psychopharmacol,* **11**, 4 suppl. S33–S37.
14. Holm KJ, Spencer CM. (1999) Reboxetine: A review of its use in depression. *CNS Drugs, 12* (1), 65–83.
15. Moll E, Neumann N, Schmid-Burgk W, *et al.* (1994) Safety and efficacy during long-term treatment with moclobemide. *Clin Neuropharmacol,* **17**, suppl 1, S74–S87.
16. Hilton S, Jaber B, Ruch R. (1995) Moclobemide safety: Monitoring a newly developed product in the 1990s.
17. Robinson DS, Roberts LD, Smith JM, *et al.* (1996) The safety profile of Nefazodone. *J Clin Psychiatry,* **57**, suppl 2, 31–38

Antidepressant-induced hyponatraemia

Most antidepressants have been associated with hyponatraemia. The mechanism of this adverse effect is probably the syndrome of inappropriate secretion of anti-diuretic syndrome (SIADH). Hyponatraemia is a rare but potentially serious adverse effect of antidepressants, which demands careful monitoring, particularly of those patients at greatest risk of hyponatraemia.

✦ **Risk factors**

> **History of hyponatraemia**
> **Extreme old age (> 80 years)**
> **Diuretics**
> **Diabetes mellitus**
> **Hypertension**
> **Reduced renal function**
> **COAD**

✦ **Monitoring**

i) **Patients with no risk factors**

No monitoring required, but serum sodium measurements should be undertaken when hyponatraemia is suspected.

> *Symptoms of hyponatraemia include lethargy, confusion, nausea, muscle cramps and seizures.*

ii) **Patients with at least one risk factor**

* ❖ Baseline urea and electrolytes (U&Es)
* ❖ *Monthly* U&Es for 3 months
* ❖ U&Es every 3–6 months thereafter
* ❖ *Immediate* serum sodium determination for any patients showing signs of confusion or lethargy or if seizures occur.

✦ **Remedial actions when hyponatraemia occurs**

> **Withdraw antidepressant immediately**
>
> If serum **sodium >125mmol/L**, monitor serum sodium daily until concentration is above 135mmol/L.
>
> If serum **sodium is <125mmol/L**, refer immediately to specialist medical care.

♦ **Re-starting antidepressant therapy**

i)   Consider ECT (which is *not* linked to hyponatraemia)

ii)   Give a drug from a different class but note that it is likely that all antidepressants cause hyponatraemia. Begin with a low dose, increase slowly and monitor closely, as described above.

References

Blass DM, Pearson VE. (2000) SIADH with multiple antidepressants in a geriatric patient. *J Clin Psychiatry*, **61**, 448–449 (letter).

McAskill R, Taylor D. (1997) Psychotropics and hyponatraemia. *Psych Bull*, **21**, 33–35.

Sharma H, Pompei P. (1996) Antidepressant-induced hyponatraemia in the aged: avoidance and management strategies. *Drugs Aging*, **8**, 430–435.

Strachan J, Shepherd J. (1998) Hyponatraemia associated with the use of selective serotonin re-uptake inhibitors. *Australian NZ J Psychiatry*, **32**, 295–298.

ECT and psychotropics

There have been few well-controlled studies on the use of psychotropics in ECT and much of the information available is based on clinical experience or anecdotal reports. For drugs known to lower seizure threshold it is best to start treatment with a low stimulus (50mC). Staff should be alerted to the possibility of prolonged seizures and I/V diazepam should be available. Orientation and cognitive function should be monitored in all patients after ECT. Information contained in the table below is based on The Second Report of the Royal College of Psychiatrists' Special Committee on ECT.

Drug	Effect on ECT seizure duration	Comment
Benzodiazepines	↓	If possible avoid during ECT, as these will raise the seizure threshold. This includes short-acting benzos for night sedation. Those on long-term therapy should have their dosage slowly reduced and/or tapered off if clinically indicated–and if practicable–before ECT. If sedation required, consider the use of hydroxyzine.
Selective serotonin reuptake inhibitors (SSRIs)	? ↑	Despite anecdotal reports suggesting a problem, studies indicate taking SSRIs during ECT is safe. If clinically indicated, there is no contraindication to continuing SSRIs during ECT.
Tricyclic antidepressants (TCAs)	? ↑	No studies looking at seizure duration with TCAs during ECT but TCAs can lower seizure threshold. As some elderly patients experience asystole after ECT, it is best to avoid TCAs in elderly and those with cardiac disease. TCAs may be safely continued during ECT. Abrupt withdrawal prior to ECT is not advisable. Monitor hypotensive effects. Anticholinergic effects may predispose to confusion.
Monoamine oxidase inhibitors (MAOIs)	? –	Little information about effect on seizure threshold and few studies of use in ECT. Monitor hypotensive effects. Do not need to discontinue but _do inform anaesthetist_. No information at this time on moclobemide and ECT, although manufacturer recommends stopping it 24 hours before ECT.
Lithium	? ↑	Literature on lithium and ECT is conflicting. One retrospective study demonstrated more cognitive problems with lithium/ECT vs ECT alone. However, two prospective studies found no such problems. Although some sources recommend stopping lithium 48 hours prior to treatment, it need not be stopped if a low stimulus is used at the start of therapy and the patient is monitored closely throughout treatment for cognitive effects and evidence of lithium toxicity.
Barbiturates	↓	All barbiturates may shorten seizure duration and methohexital and thiopental have been reported to induce cardiac arrythmias. Nonetheless, barbiturates are frequently used for narcosis during ECT, but it is recommended that low to moderate doses be used.
Antipsychotics	? ↑	Few studies on antipsychotics and ECT. There are some reports of augmentation of effect when used for schizophrenia. Manufacturers recommend clozapine is suspended for 24 hours prior to ECT but safe concurrent use has been reported. Anticholinergic effects may predispose to confusion and augment effects of atropine-like pre/post-meds. May also increase risk of hypotension.
Anticonvulsants	↓	Continue during ECT if prescribed as mood stabiliser but may need higher energy stimulus. If used for epilepsy, their effect should be to normalise seizure threshold.

References

1. Bazire S. (ed). (1999) *Psychotropic Drug Directory*. Quay Books Division, Dinton, Wilts.
2. Curran S, Freeman CP. (1995) ECT and drugs. (In) Freeman, CP (ed). *The ECT Handbook – The second report of the Royal College of Psychiatrists' special committee on ECT*. Henry Ling Ltd, Dorset Press.
3. Jarvis MR, Goewert AJ, Zorumski CF. (1992) Novel antidepressants and maintenance electroconvulsive therapy. *Ann Clin Psychiatry*, **4**, 275–284.
4. Kellner CH, Nixon DW, Bernstein HJ. (1991) ECT – Drug interactions: a review. *Psychopharmacol Bull*, **27**, 595–609.
5. Maidment I. (1997) The interaction between psychiatric medicines and ECT. *Hospital Pharmacist* **4**, 102–105.
6. Welch CA. Electroconvulsive therapy. (In) Ciraulo DA, Shader, RI, Greenblatt, DJ, Creelman W. (ed). (1995) *Drug Interactions in Psychiatry – 2nd edition*. Williams & Wilkins.

Treatment of acute mania or hypomania

Step 1

❖   **Begin or optimise mood stabilisers***

Lithium	0.6–1.2mmol/L
Carbamazepine	8–12mg/L[1]
Valproate	50–100mg/L[1]

❖   Withdraw all antidepressants immediately[2]

Step 2
(usually necessary and advisable for all patients)

❖   **Begin benzodiazepine****

Lorazepam	1mg tds[3]
Clonazepam	1mg bd[4]

Evaluate over 2–3 days
Withdraw after resolution of symptoms

Step 3
(only if steps 1 and 2 are ineffective)

❖   **Begin antipsychotic*****

Haloperidol	5mg tds[2]
Chlorpromazine	100mg tds[2]
Olanzapine	10mg OD[5]

Evaluate over 1–2 weeks
Withdraw after resolution of symptoms[6]

Step 4
(last resort)

❖   **Consider other putative antimanic agents**
e.g.
Combination of mood stabilisers[2]

Lamotrigine[7]	– dosing as for epilepsy
Gabapentin[8]	– begin at 300mg/day, increasing to 2,400mg/day
Clozapine[9,10]	– dosing as for schizophrenia
Risperidone[11]	– up to 6mg/day

*   Suggested *starting* doses:
Lithium   400mg MR OD
Carbamazepine   200mg MR BD
Valproate   500mg MR OD

**   Doses recommended are for initiation of therapy.
Many centres use higher doses where necessary.
e.g. lorazepam up to 8mg/day; clonazepam up to 8mg/day

*** Some centres begin antipsychotic medication at an earlier stage, especially if psychosis is present.

References

1. Taylor DM, Duncan D. (1997) Doses of carbamazepine and valproate in bipolar affective disorder. *Psych Bull,* **21**, 221–223.
2. American Psychiatric Association. (1994) Practice guideline for the treatment of patients with bipolar disorder. *Am J Psychiatry,* **151**, 1–36.
3. Modell JG, Lenox RH, Weiner S. (1985) Inpatient clinical trial of lorazepam for the management of manic agitation. *J Clin Psychopharmacol,* **5**, 109–113.
4. Sachs GS, Rosenbaum JF, Jones J. (1990) Adjunctive clonazepam for maintenance treatment of bipolar affective disorder. *J Clin Psychopharmacol,* **10**, 42–47.
5. Tohen M, Sanger TM, McElroy SL, *et al.* (1999) Olanzapine versus placebo in the treatment of acute mania. *Am J Psychiatry,* **156**, 702–709.
6. Soares JC, Mallinger AG, Gershon S. (1997) The role of antipsychotic agents in the treatment of bipolar disorder patients. *Int Clin Psychopharmacol,* **12**, 65–76.
7. Calabrese JR, Bowden CL, McElroy SL, *et al.* (1999) Spectrum of activity of lamotrigine in treatment-refractory bipolar disorder. *Am J Psychiatry,* **156**, 1019–1023.
8. Cabras PL, Hardoy MJ, Hardoy MC, *et al.* (1999) Clinical experience with gabapentin in patients with bipolar or schizoaffective disorder: results of an open-label study. *J Clin Psychiatry,* **60**, 245–248.
9. Mahmood T, Devlin M, Silverstone T. (1997) Clozapine in the management of bipolar and schizoaffective manic episodes resistant to standard treatment. *Australian NZ J Psychiatry,* **31**, 424–426.
10. Green AI, Tohen M, Patel JK, *et al.* (2000) Clozapine in the treatment of refractory psychotic mania. *Am J Psychiatry,* **157**, 982–986.
11. Jacobsen FM. (1995) Risperidone in the treatment of affective illness and obsessive-compulsive disorder. *J Clin Psychiatry,* **56**, 423–429.

Name	Details	Psychiatric indications (* not CSM approved)	Dose
Lithium	Inhibits the enzyme inositol-1-phosphatase → ↑ cellular responses linked to PI 2nd messenger system 1/2 life: 20hrs Renal excretion, no metabolism	Acute mania Prophylaxis of bipolar disorder Adjunctive treatment in resistant depression Schizoaffective disorder Violent patients (also with mental handicap)	Start on low (400mg) dose Serum concs to be monitored every 5 to 7 days until level is between 0.6–1.0mmol/L Thereafter check levels every 2–3 months NB. all samples must be taken 12 hours post dose
Carbamazepine	Possible peripheral benzodiazepine receptor agonist (located on GABA$_A$ receptor complex). GABA principal inhibitory peptide in brain. Peripheral benzodiazepine receptor regulates Ca^{++} channel function. ? Stops kindling process 1/2 life: 12–17 hours Metabolised by liver & then excreted by kidney Metabolite has ? some activity	Prophylaxis of bipolar illness * Rapid Cycling. (both indications- alone or in combination with Li$^+$) * Acute mania * Aggression	Usual starting-dose 200mg BD, slowly increased until dose 600–1,000mg/day is achieved. MR prep possibly better tolerated Target range for psychiatric: 8–12mg/L Sample at trough Induces own metabolism: monitor every two weeks until stable then every 3–6 months

ilising agents

Precautions	Contraindications	Side effects	Drug interactions
1. Renal function: U&E before commencing Li⁺. Excreted through kidney exclusively: potentially nephrotoxic. Change in body salt concentration can affect levels 2. 3–4% develop hypothyroidism: TFT before starting & six-monthly intervals. 3. Lithium toxicity > levels 1.5mmol/L 4. Baseline ECG Should get Li⁺ card from pharmacy	Pregnancy – consult Drug Information Service Breast-feeding – avoid Renal impairment (may be given if close monitoring practicable) Thyroidopathies Sick Sinus Syndrome	Thirst, polyuria GI upset Tremor (may treat with propranolol) Diabetes insipidus – may inhibit ADH (must maintain fluid intake) Acne Muscular weakness Cardiac arrhythmias Weight gain common (? related to thirst & intake of high calorie drinks) Hypothyroidism	**Antipsychotics** – all antipsychotics may increase lithium's neurotoxicity **Diuretics** (thiazides): increase Li⁺ concentration **ACE inhibitors**: toxicity **Diltiazem/Verapamil**: neurotoxicity **Xanthines**: increase Li⁺ excretion **NaCl**: increases Li⁺ excretion **Alcohol**: increases peak Li⁺ concentration **NSAIDs**: all cause toxicity except aspirin & sulindac. Low dose ibuprofen usually safe
1. Warn about fever, infections etc: Need pre + regular FBCs every 2 weeks for 1st 2 months. Early leucopenias usually transient and benign 2. Carbamazepine toxicity: diplopia, ataxia, sedation	Pregnancy – consult Drug Information Service Breast-feeding Possibly alcohol abuse, glaucoma, diabetes	Drowsiness, ataxia, diplopia, nausea Agranulocytosis – 1 in 20,000 Aplastic anaemia – 1 in 20,000 Transient leucopenias in approx. 10% in 1st 2 months Hypersensitivity-hepatitis SIADH Rashes – may be serious Toxic epidermal necrolysis in 1 in 20,000, monitor carefully for 2–3 months	**Antipsychotics**: may cause CNS effects (drowsiness, ataxia etc.) **Lithium**: CNS effects and increased risk of side effects of both drugs **Ca⁺⁺ channel blockers**: CNS effects **MAOIs**: Need 2 weeks washout ↓ **TCA/ neuroleptic** ?Toxicity with '**Flu Vaccine**' Enzyme inducer: affects many others including **phenytoin** and oral contraceptives

Name	Details	Psychiatric indications (* not CSM approved)	Dose
Sodium Valproate	↓ catabolism of γ - aminobutyric acid 1/2 life of 8 hours Metabolised	In cases of failure with lithium or carbamazepine: Acute mania – especially mixed affective states * Prophylaxis of manic and depressive episodes	Commence on 500mg MR daily Then increase until plasma levels reach 50–100mg/L Trough samples required MR prep may be given once daily
Clonazepam	Rapidly Absorbed: No major metabolites 1/2 life: 34 hours	* Acute mania * Adjunctive therapy with lithium in prophylaxis of bipolar disorder	1mg initially at night, ↑to 4-8mg/day over 4 weeks (divided doses)
Verapamil (Nimodipine)	Ca⁺⁺ channel blocker-inhibits Ca⁺⁺ dependent intra-cellular protein kinases 1/2 life: 5-12 hours	In cases of failure with lithium or carbamazepine: * Acute mania * Prophylaxis of bipolar disorder * Rapid cycling	40mg TDS initially, up to 80–120mg TDS (slow increase) MR preps may aid compliance Nimodipine – 60mg tds
Lamotrigine	1/2 life: 20-24 hours but 1/2 life increased by valproate and decreased by enzyme inducers	In cases of failure with lithium, carbamazepine or valproate * Acute mania * Prophylaxis of bipolar disorder * Rapid cycling	Dose as mood stabilizer not certain, likely similar to that used in epilepsy. As dose depends on concomitant medication, see Manufacturer's information

Precautions	Contraindications	Possible side effects	Drug interactions
1. Check renal & hepatic function regularly (including baseline) 2. FBC regularly	Pregnancy – consult Drug Information Service Breast-feeding Hepatic disease	Commonly: Nausea, vomiting Sedation Rarely: Ataxia Headache Anxiety Thrombocytopenia & platelet dysfunction Pancreatitis	Complex interactions with other **anticonvulsants**: need to consult neurologist or Drug Information Potentiates activity of **aspirin & warfarin** May increase **MAOI & TCA** levels
1. Check hepatic & renal function regularly 2. FBC regularly 3. Avoid sudden withdrawal	Respiratory depression Porphyria	Commonly: Drowsiness, Fatigue, Dizziness, Muscle Hypotonia	Ataxia & dysarthria possibly with **lithium** or **antipsychotics** Additive CNS depressant effects Increased levels of **phenytoin**
1. Monitor BP, pulse 2. Monitor ECG 3. Elderly	Conduction defects (myocardial) Pregnancy Breast-feeding Cardiac failure	Hypotension, Bradycardia, AV block, G I Symptoms – constipation very common with verapamil, rare with nimodipine	Neurotoxicity with **lithium** or **carbamazepine** Other **hypotensives** **Antiarrhythmics** **Digoxin** **Beta-blockers** – can be fatal with verapamil
1. Monitor patient for rash – more likely to occur in children, with concomitant valproate or if dose started too high or increased too quickly. Most rashes occur within 8 weeks of starting therapy	Pregnancy – consult Drug Information Service Hepatic impairment	Rash, Ataxia, Diplopia, Headache, Vomiting	**Valproate** increases levels of lamotrigine Lamotrigine may increase levels of the **carbamazepine epoxide metabolite**

Algorithm for the treatment of rapid-cycling bipolar affective disorder

1st line		**Lithium**
	or	**Carbamazepine**
	or	**Valproate**
2nd line		**Combine two or more first line drugs**
3rd line		**Add thyroxine** *(to double free thyroid levels)*
4th line		**Withdraw thyroxine** **add nimodipine** *(30-60mg tds)*
5th line		**Withdraw nimodipine** **add clozapine**

Notes

✧ Rapid cycling = more than four episodes of (hypo)mania/depression in a 12 month period

✧ Take a detailed history and consider precipitants of mood change which might be predicted or controlled (e.g. external stressors, life events and changes during menstrual cycle).

✧ Target plasma levels (at trough) are:
Lithium   0.6–1.0mmol/L
Carbamazepine   8–12mg/L
Valproate   50–100mg/L

✧ Clozapine is not licensed for use in bipolar disorder. Do not use with carbamazepine.

✧ Other neuroleptics may be used but should usually be reserved for 'acute' treatment of hypomanic symptoms. Continuous therapy is not recommended because of long-term adverse effects such as tardive dyskinesia.

✧ Lamotrigine may be effective but few data at present.

References

Calabrese JR, Meltzer HY, Markovitz PJ. (1991) Clozapine prophylaxis in rapid cycling bipolar disorder. *J Clin Psychopharmacol*, **11**, 396–397.

Calabrese JR, Woyshville, MJ. (1995) A medication algorithm for treatment of bipolar rapid cycling? *Clin Psychiatry*, **56** [suppl 3], 11–18.

Duncan D, McConnell HW, Taylor D. (1998) Lamotrigine in bipolar affective disorder. *Psych Bull*, **22**, 630–632.

Goodnick PJ. (1995) Nimodipine treatment of rapid cycling bipolar disorder. *J Clin Psychiatry*, **56**, 330.

McConnell HW, Duncan D. (1998a) *Behavioural effects of antiepileptic drugs*. In: Psychiatric co-morbidity in epilepsy: basic mechanisms, diagnosis and treatment. McConnell HW and Snyder PJ (eds.) American Psychiatric Press, Washington D.C., pg. 205–244.

McConnell HW and Duncan D. *The Use of Antiepileptic Drugs in Psychiatry*. In Kerwin R. (ed): The Maudsley Textbook of Psychiatry (in press).

McElroy SL, Keck Jr PE, Pope Jr HG, *et al.* (1988) Valproate in the treatment of rapid cycling bipolar disorder. *J Clin Psychopharmacol*, **8**, 275–279.

Pazzagila PJ, Post RM, Ketter TA, *et al.* (1993) Preliminary controlled trial of nimodipine in ultra-rapid cycling affective dysregulation. *Psychiatry Research*, **49**, 257–272.

Taylor DM, Duncan D. (1996) Treatment options for rapid-cycling bipolar affective disorder. *Psych Bull*, **20**, 601–603.

Taylor DM, Duncan D. (1997) Doses of carbamazepine and valproate in bipolar affective disorder. *Psych Bull*, **21**, 221–223.

IV

Treatment of

Anxiety

Treatment of anxiety disorders

The treatment of first choice for anxiety disorders is cognitive behaviour therapy (CBT).[1-3] Patient choice and availability of an appropriately trained therapist may sometimes dictate the choice of treatment. With limited availability of treatment, other options may include computer-aided or self-help manuals in CBT.

Pharmacotherapy for an anxiety disorder is recommended usually in combination with CBT when (a) there is co-morbidity such as depression, (b) there is failure of treatment by CBT alone, or (c) when symptoms are severely handicapping. Failure to respond should provoke a review of the diagnosis and exclusion of an organic anxiety state (e.g. thyrotoxicosis) and an examination of lifestyle factors (e.g. excessive caffeine or recreational drugs).

Specific phobia

First choice therapy is graded self-exposure and cessation of safety behaviours. Treatment of specific phobia of blood or injury may gain added benefit from exposure combined with 'applied tension'.[4]

Pharmacotherapy is not indicated except in one-off circumstances (for example use of a benzodiazepine for a severe flying phobia).

Panic disorder and agoraphobia

First choice: CBT (graded self-exposure or cognitive therapy and behavioural experiments to test out the catastrophic beliefs and dropping of safety behaviours).

Second choice: if failure of CBT or significant co-morbidity, then an SSRI is the first line pharmacological treatment.[5] There are no trials comparing different SSRIs, which are probably all equally effective. Doses are: paroxetine, (starting dose 10mg gradually increased up to 40mg), fluvoxamine (25–200mg), citalopram (10–40mg), sertraline (25–150mg) or fluoxetine (10–60mg). The onset of action may take may not appear for six weeks and the full response may take up to 12 weeks.

✦ Up to 40% of patients with panic disorder experience an 'activation syndrome' of agitation on commencing an SSRI. This can be minimised by education, using a half or even quarter the starting dose than that used for depression and gradually increasing the dose. Fluoxetine might have a greater association with an activation syndrome and is not usually recommended for panic disorder.[5]

✦ About 40% of patients relapse on discontinuation of an SSRI and so treatment is usually continued for a minimum of 12 months. Once in remission then the dose may be reduced slowly.

✦ Discontinuation symptoms may occur especially with shorter acting SSRIs such as paroxetine. Once in remission, the dose should therefore be tapered slowly (e.g. 25% every 2 months) or if necessary replaced by a longer acting SSRI (e.g. fluoxetine or citalopram).

Alternatives

Opinions differ as to the order of alternative options if failure of an SSRI. The options include:

✦ A second SSRI or a tricyclic antidepressant (e.g. imipramine starting dose 25mg gradually increased to 250mg daily or clomipramine 25 to 250mg daily). Tricyclics are often poorly tolerated because of anticholinergic side effects or problems with weight gain. A low starting dose should be used and the dose gradually increased.

✦ An irreversible MAOI (e.g. phenelzine 45–90mg daily) or a RIMA (e.g. moclobemide 300–600mg daily). Allow at least two weeks between discontinuing an SSRI or tricyclic (five weeks if fluoxetine) before commencing a MAOI or RIMA.

✦ A benzodiazepine (e.g. alprazolam (2–6mg daily) or clonazepam (1–2mg) daily or diazepam (5–40mg daily)) is often prescribed in the USA. Benzodiazepines tend to be associated with improvements within the first week, but tolerance usually limits their use in the longer term. They are therefore sometimes used in addition to an SSRI to gain short-term benefits and ameliorate an activation syndrome. Adverse effects can include sedation, fatigue, memory disturbances, ataxia and slurred speech. Benzodiazepines are also likely to produce withdrawal symptoms. If used with an SSRI, a planned discontinuation and gradual tapering should occur within six weeks. If a benzodiazepine is used alone then there is a high risk of relapse when it is discontinued. Shorter acting benzodiazepines (such as alprazolam and clonazepam) cause inter-dose rebound anxiety (requiring multiple daily dosing of two to three times a day). Patients often have difficulty tapering the last dose and their use for panic disorder is therefore recommended only if combined with an SSRI and in the short term. They should not be used in patients with suicidal ideation or a history of alcohol or substance abuse.

Specific or non-generalised social phobia

First choice: CBT (Graded exposure and/or cognitive therapy and behavioural experiments (to test out beliefs) and dropping of safety behaviours).

Second choice: Beta-blockers (e.g. propranolol starting dose 20mg gradually increased up to 60mg or atenolol 50–100mg) may be helpful in performance anxiety (for example public speaking or a musical performance) or non-generalised social phobia.[6]

Alternatives: Treat as for generalised social phobia.

Generalised social phobia or social anxiety disorder

First choice: CBT (Graded exposure and/or cognitive therapy and behavioural experiments (to test out beliefs) and dropping of safety behaviours).

Second choice: If failure of CBT or significant co-morbidity, then use an SSRI (paroxetine starting dose 20mg gradually increased up to 50mg, fluoxetine 20–60mg, fluvoxamine 50–150mg, sertraline 50–150mg, citalopram 20–50mg). Those with social phobia do not usually experience an activation syndrome (as in panic disorder) and can usually commence on a normal starting dose of an SSRI. The starting dose is used for two to four weeks and then increased as necessary.

✦ The onset of action is usually within six weeks and an adequate trial is eight weeks. The full response may take up to 12 weeks to appear.

✦ About 40% of patients relapse on discontinuation of an SSRI and so treatment is usually continued for a minimum of 12 months. Once in remission then the dose may be reduced slowly.

✦ Discontinuation symptoms occur especially with shorter acting SSRIs such as paroxetine. The dose should therefore be tapered slowly (e.g. 25% every two months) or use a longer acting SSRI.

Alternatives:

✦ If failure of an SSRI then switch to an MAOI (e.g. phenelzine 45–90mg daily) or a RIMA (e.g. moclobemide 300–600mg daily). Allow at least two weeks between discontinuing an SSRI (five weeks if fluoxetine) before commencing a MAOI or RIMA.

✦ Beta-blockers (e.g. propranolol starting dose 20mg gradually increased up to 60mg or atenolol 50–100mg) may be useful to augment the response to an SSRI or MAOI.

✦ Clonidine may be helpful to augment the response for symptoms of blushing.

✦ Benzodiazepines such as clonazepam (2–6mg daily) or alprazolam (2–6mg daily) are sometimes prescribed in the USA for social phobia. However continuous use is likely to produce a high risk of tolerance, relapse and withdrawal symptoms on discontinuation. Side effects at higher dose may include sedation, forgetfulness, impaired concentration and disinhibition especially when used intermittently. The use of benzodiazepines for social phobia is not therefore recommended in the UK unless patients have failed previous treatments. Benzodiazepines are especially not recommended in patients with co-morbidity of depression or a history of alcohol or substance abuse.

Generalised Anxiety Disorder

First choice: CBT (anxiety management training and cognitive therapy).

Second choice: If failure of CBT or significant co-morbidity, then use an SSRI or SNRI starting in a low dose (similar to treatment of panic disorder).

Alternatives:

✦ Buspirone (starting dose 15mg daily gradually increased up to 60mg daily). Allow at least two to four weeks to have modest benefit in symptoms. There is no potential for dependence.

✦ Benzodiazepines with a long half-life (e.g. diazepam 2–30mg daily). There is potential for dependence especially in personality disorder, where there is poor impulse control or a history of substance abuse. Benzodiazepines are normally restricted to maximum of four weeks continuously and to taper the dose accordingly. Continuous low dose prescribing may however be justified in some treatment-resistant patients.

Post-traumatic stress disorder

First choice: CBT (Imaginal exposure, graded self-exposure and/or cognitive therapy for beliefs about the symptoms or the trauma and dropping of excessive safety behaviours.)

Second choice: If failure of CBT or significant co-morbidity, treat as for panic disorder and agoraphobia initially with an SSRI or nefazodone or venlafaxine.[2]

Alternatives

✦ If failure of one class, then switch to a MAOI or a RIMA although there are mixed reports of efficacy. Allow at least two weeks between discontinuing an SSRI (five weeks if fluoxetine) before commencing a MAOI or RIMA.

✦ In treatment-resistant cases, open trials suggest an anti-convulsant (carbamazepine[7] or valproic acid[8]) may be of benefit.

✦ An alpha$_2$ agonist (clonidine 0.2–0.4mg daily) or a beta-blocker in high doses may be useful for hyper-arousal symptoms.

✦ The role of benzodiazepines is very limited and might pose a special problem for patients with PTSD in discontinuation.

Obsessive Compulsive Disorder (OCD)

First choice: CBT (graded self-exposure and response prevention and/or cognitive therapy). In treatment-resistant cases, patients may benefit from a more intensive programme as an in-patient.

Second choice: If failure of CBT or significant co-morbidity or severely handicapping, then a serotonin reuptake inhibitor (SRI) is the treatment of choice preferably in combination with CBT (fluoxetine at a starting dose of 20mg gradually increasing up to 80mg, paroxetine 20–60mg, sertraline 50–200mg, fluvoxamine 50–300mg, citalopram 20–60mg, or clomipramine 50–275mg).[3–9] All SRIs are probably equally effective and the choice depends upon the side effect profile. Gradually increase the dose to the maximum tolerated within six to eight weeks of the start of treatment.

✦ An adequate trial of an SRI must include the maximum tolerated dose for a duration of 12 weeks before changing to an alternative SRI or augmenting. Blood level monitoring of clomipramine might be required for higher doses of clomipramine. ECG monitoring is also highly recommended.

✦ Maintenance treatment with an SRI should be for a minimum of a year. In maintenance treatment, drug dosages can be reduced up to 50% of that used in acute episode without a significant reduction in symptoms.
   a) Patients who have taken an SRI are at a high risk of relapse when treatment is stopped and of discontinuation symptoms (especially within the first two months and if withdrawal is abrupt). Discontinuation of a SRI in OCD should therefore be tapered slowly (e.g. 25% every two months).
   b) Some patients are extra sensitive to commencing on an SSRI and may need to begin on a dose 1–2mg fluoxetine or paroxetine as an elixir and the dose very gradually increased.
   c) Children and adolescents with OCD may also be safely treated with an SSRI. A paediatric subtype of OCD characterised by pre-pubertal onset and episodic nature has been associated with a group A beta haemolytic streptococci pharyngitis that triggers an autoimmune response. This may be best treated by dialysis.

✦ If failure of an SRI, switch to an alternative SSRI or clomipramine.

✦ If failure of at least two SSRIs and clomipramine, then augment with a low dose of a neu-roleptic (e.g. haloperidol 0.5mg)[10] or an atypical neuroleptic (risperidone 1mg a day)[11] especially when there is a co-morbid tic disorder. There are also reports of exacerbation of OCD in some patients with an atypical anti-psychotic when used alone without an SSRI.

✦ In treatment refractory patients, opinions vary as to the order of various options described in the literature. An adequate trial of an augmenting agent is at least eight weeks. Options include:
Mega-doses of an SSRI.[12,13]
Intra-venous clomipramine[14] or citalopram followed by a higher oral dose.
An SNRI (e.g. venlafaxine).[15]
SSRI augmentation with an atypical SRI (trazadone or nefazodone).[16]
SSRI augmentation with tramadol.
SSRI augmentation with clonazepam (1–3mg in divided doses daily).[17]
SSRI augmentation with an alternative SSRI.[18]
MAOI (phenelzine 45–90mg daily).[19] Allow at least two weeks between discontinuing an SSRI (five weeks if fluoxetine) before commencing a MAOI.
Anti-androgen therapy (cyproterone acetate).[20]

Body Dysmorphic Disorder

First choice: Cognitive behaviour therapy.

Second choice: If failure of CBT or significant co-morbidity or severe symptoms, then a SSRI is the treatment of choice in combination with CBT as for OCD.[21] Note that 'delusional' patients with BDD may respond to an SSRI just as well as 'non-delusional' patients.[22] There is no good evidence that pimozide or an antipsychotic drug by itself is of any benefit. Like OCD, a low dose of antipsychotic may be indicated as an adjunct to an SSRI in treatment resistant cases after trials of at least two SSRIs and clomipramine.

Alternative:
✦ Opiate antagonists (naltrexone up to 100–200mg daily) may be useful for skin-picking or other impulsive behaviours.[23]

Hypochondriasis

First choice: Cognitive behaviour therapy.

Second choice: If failure of CBT or significant co-morbidity or severe symptoms, then an SRI is the treatment of choice preferably in combination with CBT as for OCD.

Trichotillomania

First choice: Behaviour therapy (daily self-monitoring of hairs pulled & habit reversal)

Second choice: If failure of behaviour therapy or severe symptoms, then a SRI is the treatment of choice as for OCD.[24]

Alternatives
✦ Naltrexone alone or augmentation of an SSRI.[25]

References

1. Fawcett J, Stein D, Jobson KO. (1999) Treatment algorithms in psychopharmacology Chichester, John Wiley & Sons.
2. Foa EB, Davidson JRT, Frances A. (1999) The Expert Consensus Guideline Series: Treatment of Posttraumatic Stress Disorder. *J Clin Psychiatry* **60** (suppl 16).
3. March JS, Frances A, Kahn DA, Carpenter D. (1997) The Expert Consensus Guideline Series: Treatment of Obsessive–Compulsive Disorder. *J Clin Psychiatry* **58** (suppl 4).
4. Ost L-G, Fellenius J, Sterner U. (1991) Applied tension, exposure in vivo, and tension-only in the treatment of blood phobia. *Behav Res Ther* **29**,561–574.
5. Ballenger JC, Davidson JRT, Lecrubier Y, *et al.* (1998) Consensus Statement on Panic Disorder From the International Consensus Group on Depression and Anxiety. *J Clin Psychiatry* **59** (suppl 8), 47–54.
6. Sutherland SM, Davidson JRT. (1999) Social phobia in Textbook of treatment Algorithms in Psychopharmacology Edited by Fawcett J, Stein DJ, Jobson KO. Chichester, John Wiley & Sons.
7. Lipper S, Davidson JRT, Grady TA, *et al.* (1986) Preliminary study of carbamezepine in post-traumatic stress. Psychosomatics **27**, 849–854.
8. Fesler FA. (1991) Valproate in combat-related post-traumatic stress disorder. *J Clin Psychiatry* **52**, 361–364.
9. Jenike MA. (1998) Drug treatment of obsessive-compulsive disorders. In: Obsessive compulsive disorders: Practical Management Edited by Jenike MA, Baer L, Minichellio WE. St Louis, Mosby.
10. McDougle CJ, Goodman WK, Leckman JF. (1994) Haloperidol addition in fluvoxamine refractory obsessive-compulsive disorder. *Arch Gen Psychiatry* **51**, 302–308.
11. McDougle CJ, Fleischmann RL, Epperson CN. (1995) Risperidone addition in fluvoxamine-refractory obsessive-compulsive disorder: three cases. *J Clin Psychiatry* **56**, 526–528.
12. Bejerot S, Bodlund O. (1998) Response to a high doses of citalopram in treatment-resistant obsessive compulsive disorder. *Acta Psychiatr Scand* **98**, 423–424.
13. Byerly MJ, Goodman WK, Christensen R. (1996) High doses of sertraline for treatment resistant obsessive-compulsive disorder. *Am J Psychiatry* **153**, 1232–1233.
14. Koran LM, Sallee FR, Pallanti S. (1997) Rapid benefit of intravenous pulse loading of clomipramine in obsessive–compulsive disorder. *Am J Psychiatry* **154**, 396–401.
15. Ananth J, Burgoyne K, Smith M. (1995) Venlafaxine for the treatment of obsessive–compulsive disorder. *Am J Psychiatry* **152**, 1832.
16. Jenike MA. (1990) Approaches to the patient with treatment-refractory obsessive–compulsive disorder. *J Clin Psychiatry* **51**, 15–21.
17. Hewlett WA, Vinogradov S, Agras WS. (1992) Clomipramine, clonazepam, and clonidine treatment of obsessive–compulsive disorder. *J Clin Psychopharmacol* **12**, 420–430.
18. Markovitz PJ, Stagno SJ, Calabrese JR. (1990) Buspirone augmentation of fluoxetine on obsessive–compulsive disorder. *Am J Psychiatry* **147**, 798–800.
19. Vallejo J, Olivares J, Marcos T. (1992) Clomipramine versus phenelzine in obsessive–compulsive disorder: a controlled clinical trial. *Br J Psychiatry* **161**, 665–670.
20. Casas M, Alvarez E, Duro P. (1986) Anti-androgenic treatment of obsessive–compulsive neurosis. *Acta Psychiatr Scand* **73**, 221–222.
21. Hollander E, Allen A, Kwon J, *et al.* (1999) Clomipramine vs desipramine crossover trial in body dysmorphic disorder: selective efficacy of a serotonin reuptake inhibitor in imagined ugliness. *Arch Gen Psychiatry* **56**, 1033–1042.
22. Phillips KA, Dwight MM, McElroy SL. (1998) Efficacy and safety of fluvoxamine in body dysmorphic disorder. *J Clin Psychiatry* **59**, 165–171.
23. Kim SW. (1998) Opioid antagonists in the treatment of impulse control disorders. *J Clin Psychiatry* **54**, 159–164.
24. Keuthen NJ, O'Sullivan RL, Jefferys DE. (1998) Trichotillomania: Clinical concepts and treatment approaches. In: Obsessive compulsive disorders: Practical Management Edited by Jenike MA, Baer L, Minichellio WE.
25. Carrion VC. (1995) Naltrexone for the treatment of trichotillomania: a case report. *J Clin Psychopharmacol* **15**: 444–445.

Hypnotics

Before treating insomnia with drugs:

Take a thorough sleep history

Is the insomnia initial or middle insomnia? Is there early morning wakening? Consider whole lifetime: most 1° insomniacs have always been poor sleepers.

Determine the pattern of sleep

Is the sleep pattern normal? Has the diurnal rhythm become disturbed? Are other factors (nightwork; jet-lag) involved?

Duration of disturbance

Is the sleep disturbance chronic and stable or acute?

Look for possible causes of sleep disturbance

✦ Psychiatric illness e.g. anxiety disorder, depression, acute psychosis, mania.

✦ Drug-induced (theophylline, sympathomimetics, caffeine, nocturnal anticholinergics, tranylcypromine, etc).

✦ Drug-withdrawal in dependence (consider affect of withdrawal from therapeutic agents).

✦ Medical disorder e.g. thyroid disease, menopausal symptoms, peptic ulceration due to excessive alcohol or caffeine, any pain.

✦ Coming into hospital or other change of environment.

Think about alternative treatments

Sleep hygiene:

✦ Avoid daytime naps/resting/reading in bed; reduce caffeine intake; anxiety management; relaxation techniques. Encourage patient to go to bed at same time; reserve bed for sleep. Exercise early in the day helps but exercise late in the day is deleterious.

✦ Always treat underlying causes.

If hypnotics are to be prescribed:

✦ With nursing staff, counsel patient about the use of hypnotics: explain that they may only be used for a short time. Outline risks of tolerance, dependence and withdrawal.

General guidelines on hypnotic use:

✦ Avoid short-acting, high potency benzodiazepines e.g. lorazepam. Oxazepam is preferable. Note abuse potential of temazepam.

✦ Alternative compounds include antihistamines (e.g. promethazine), zopiclone and zolpidem.

✦ Avoid high doses.

✦ Short-term use only (no more than two weeks) with regular review; intermittent if possible.

✦ Avoid abrupt withdrawal, if use has been continuous for >2 weeks.

✦ Avoid in respiratory failure and in addiction-prone individuals.

✦ Reduce doses in the elderly.

✦ Note all antihistamines are long-acting with noticeable hangover. Some have slow onset of effect.

Benzodiazepine oral dose equivalents

Benzodiazepine	Equivalent Diazepam dose	Approximate duration of action
Diazepam	5mg	2–4 days
Chlordiazepoxide	15mg (10–25mg)	2–4 days
Clonazepam	0.5mg (0.25–2mg)	1–2 days
Lorazepam	0.5 (0.5–1mg)	8–12 hours
Nitrazepam	5mg (2.5–10mg)	12–24 hours
Oxazepam	15mg (5–30mg)	8–12 hours
Temazepam	10mg (7.5–15mg)	8 hours

Benzodiazepine oral / parenteral dose equivalents

Drug	Oral dose (mg)	Equivalent IV or IM dose (mg)
Diazepam	10	10
Lorazepam	4	4

V

Treatment of
Special Patient Populations

Treatment of childhood mental disorders

Pharmacological treatment for children with psychiatric disorder should always be considered as just one component part of a package of psychological, social and educational intervention. Sometimes (even for some cases of drug-responsive conditions such as attention deficit/hyperactivity disorder (ADHD) or Tourette disorder) a knowledge of the natural history of disorder and a suitable psychoeducational intervention can make drug therapy unnecessary.

Summary table of child psychiatric disorders in which drug treatment is indicated

Disorder	Drugs used first-line	Drugs used second-line
Psychosis	Atypical antipsychotics (risperidone, olanzapine, amisulpride)	Typical antipsychotics (haloperidol, chlorpromazine), clozapine
Hyperkinetic disorder/ADHD	Stimulants (methylphenidate, dexamphetamine)	Imipramine, clonidine
Obsessive compulsive disorder	SSRIs (sertraline, fluoxetine, paroxetine, fluvoxamine, citalopram)	Clomipramine
Tourette syndrome/tic disorders	Haloperidol, sulpiride	Pimozide, risperidone, SSRIs
Depression	SSRIs (sertraline, fluoxetine, paroxetine, citalopram)	Tricyclic antidepressants (imipramine, amitriptyline, clomipramine)

For many of the psychological disorders of childhood, medication plays only a small role, either because of the lack of efficacy of drugs for the disorders (such as mental retardation, autism, conduct disorders) or because of the availability of effective psychological treatments (eating disorders, sleep disorders, anxiety disorders, enuresis).

Experimental studies in children are ethically and practically difficult, so much of the knowledge of pharmacokinetics and pharmacodynamics has been extrapolated from adult studies. Caution is needed until appropriate efficacy and safety studies are carried out in children. For this reason, manufacturers' package inserts will often say "not recommended for children" and sometimes the licences, even of valuable and well-studied drugs, do not extend to children. This is a problem for all paediatric prescribers, not only in mental health. As a result, the psychiatrist's duty to offer the most valuable treatments to patients will often entail the recommendation of medicines beyond the terms of their licence. The commonly held idea that drugs are more hazardous in young people is not necessarily true. For example, antipsychotic-induced akathisia seems to be less common in children and adolescents (while acute dystonias are probably more common).

Drug response varies with age, weight, sex, disease-state, absorption, distribution, metabolism and excretion. For many drugs, bioavailability is lower in children due to rapid metabolism and distribution in a relatively larger extracellular fluid space; on the other hand, many will more readily cross the blood-brain barrier in children than in adults. Titration of dosage within a mg/kg range is therefore the rule, since strict adherence to a single dose will undertreat some children and overtreat others.

Hyperkinetic disorder and ADHD

Children who meet the ICD–10 criteria for hyperkinetic disorder (HD) should have a treatment plan that includes the reduction of hyperactive behaviour as one of the goals. It is not the only goal: it will also be important to detect and treat any coexisting disorders, to prevent the development of conduct disorder (or reduce it if it has developed), to promote academic and social learning, improve emotional adjustment and self-esteem and relieve family distress. A multimodal treatment approach will usually be needed. Behaviour therapy has some effect in reducing hyperactivity and promoting organised and attentive behaviour; but the treatment effect in trials is less than that of stimulant medication. Stimulants should therefore be considered for children over four years when advice to family and school and simple behavioural management have not resolved the problem. They should only be prescribed after a child mental health evaluation has established the indication. Once the treatment is established, however, routine prescribing and monitoring can reasonably be carried out within primary care.

For children with lesser degrees of hyperactivity—i.e. those with a DSM-IV diagnosis of Attention Deficit/Hyperactivity(ADHD), falling short of the more severe condition of hyperkinetic disorder—underlying causes such as learning disabilities, hearing impairment, family stresses, attachment disruptions and emotional disorders, should be carefully sought. Indications for medication in this group will usually arise only if the problems have not resolved with approaches designed to remove environmental causes or treat psychologically. There may be a temptation to rely unduly on the effect of medication and to use for mild cases where educational intervention and psychological treatment would be sufficient.

Prescription of stimulants

Methylphenidate and dexamphetamine are the only drugs licensed in the UK for the treatment of hyperactivity. There is a large evidence base, with many controlled trials asserting their value as an effective therapy with few hazards. The use of non-licensed drugs, or polypharmacy, should be on the advice of a specialist. Both stimulants have broadly similar effects on children's behaviour: they reduce hyperactive behaviour, enhance several aspects of information processing and increase on-task attentiveness.

Initial medication should be as a trial. Placebo control is not routinely necessary but helps in problem cases. Medication should be discussed and explained with the child, parents and teachers before it is started. While medication is being started, the family will need quick and ready access to the prescriber to report progress and any adverse effects. Methylphenidate will usually be the first choice. If titration of methylphenidate (see below) does not produce a clinically satisfactory response, then dexamphetamine should be prescribed. Pemoline has been used in the past but is now withdrawn from the market because of toxicity and is available only on a named patient basis in the UK.

The usual starting dose of methylphenidate is 5.0mg (dexamphetamine 2.5mg) twice daily with the dose being adjusted in the light of response. The dose may need to rise as high as 20mg with breakfast, 20mg in the late morning or early afternoon, and 10mg in late afternoon. If a dose range higher than that is contemplated, then more intensive monitoring should be used and a specialist consulted. Several doses a day are usually needed. Psychological action has a peak in the first hour and the effect wanes rapidly, with little action after about four hours. Accordingly, most children will be losing the effect of a breakfast dose by midday. Subsequent doses may then have to be given at school. Methylphenidate slow release tablets are available in some countries and can be provided in the UK on a named patient basis.

Monitoring

Psychological response should be monitored with rating scales of behaviours (e.g. Conners abbreviated scale) completed regularly and systematically in different settings—e.g. by parents and school. Re-evaluation at the clinic should be carried out when rating scales suggest a therapeutic response is being achieved, or if there is no response after a month of therapy. Physical monitoring should include the plotting of height and weight along standardised growth curves, and examination for the appearance of any tics. Adverse psychological effects such as lack of spontaneity, depression and excessive perseveration should be assessed specifically, with ratings, interview and observational methods. Questioning should elicit any difficulties in getting to sleep, appetite disturbance, stomach-aches, headaches and dizziness. Many of the adverse effects of stimulants are transient and decrease with time.

The long-term aim is to maintain medication until the child's maturation and learning of cognitive skills make medication unnecessary. Periodically, approximately annually, there should be a gradual withdrawal of medication over a period of two weeks to assess whether there is indeed a continuing need for medication. Drug holidays—e.g. during weekends and vacations from school—are not required routinely unless the child's growth has been affected by medication.

Unlicensed drugs

If stimulants are ineffective despite careful dose titration, or if adverse effects make them inappropriate, or if there are relative contraindications (such as tics or mood disorders), then specialist clinical review may lead to the prescription of second-line therapies. **Tricyclic antidepressants** have been shown to be more effective than placebo in randomised blinded controlled trials. The dose (approx. 1mg imipramine/kg body weight) is less than that for treating depression and the onset is quicker, usually in the first three days of treatment. The serious hazards are for the cardiovascular system: there can be tachycardia and deterioration of the ECG even years after the start of the treatment. A few cases of sudden death, presumably due to cardiac arrhythmia, have been reported in children using desipramine. Repeated ECGs and blood estimations (monthly at the start of treatment, quarterly after six months) are needed with doses over 50mg daily of imipramine. Female patients seem to reach higher blood levels with the same weight-adjusted dose than male patients, and also show more side effects. The blood level is unpredictably increased if methylphenidate is given simultaneously, so the combination should be given, if at all, only with close monitoring of blood level and ECG. In adolescents self-injury and overdose are quite common, so special care is needed and a good relationship between physician, parents and child is required.

Clonidine has some effect in reducing hyperactive behaviour, though little benefit on cognitive performance can be expected. It does not worsen tics, and may even improve them.

Low-dose **haloperidol** reduces hyperactivity through a different mechanism from the stimulants and may be effective when they fail; but dystonias can appear in children even at these very low doses so it should be regarded as a treatment of last resort. Risperidone has not undergone formal trials but is a safer alternative, though weight gain is a common hazard. New and promising drugs such as moclobemide are still under evaluation.

Stimulants in younger children and adults

Methylphenidate is officially not recommended below the age of six, though it is hard to see why the manufacturers have taken this line given the scientific evidence. Dexamphetamine is licensed down to the age of three years. Clinicians should diagnose and treat hyperkinetic disorders from the age of four years, but should do so with some caution, remembering the difficulties of diagnosis in this age group and the possibility that oppositional and noncompliant behaviour may be mislabelled as attention deficit.

Stimulants have been tried in adults presenting with ADHD, and trial evidence (though not conclusive) gives support to their use. They should only be considered when there is both a childhood history of ADHD (preferably supported by contemporary evidence such as school reports or parental recall) and the current presentation includes high levels of inattentiveness and impulsiveness. Antisocial behaviour or occupational failure may be a complication of ADHD, but are unlikely to be helped by stimulants if the core symptoms of inattentiveness and impulsiveness have disappeared.

Depression in children

Major depressive disorders in childhood should be seen as serious psychiatric conditions that may become chronic or relapsing illness. Treatment of depression includes effective resolution of the current episode and effective prophylaxis to prevent further episodes or to reduce their morbidity if they do occur. Medication should be used in conjunction with interventions designed to improve interpersonal, social and academic functioning. Cognitive behavioural therapy, interpersonal psychotherapy, counselling and other non-pharmacological approaches are all useful in this population

The trial evidence is not conclusive, but suggests that SSRIs are effective in child and adolescent depression, and should generally be the first choice of drug. Commonly used SSRIs include fluoxetine and paroxetine (which both have liquid formulations), and there is accumulating experience with sertraline and fluvoxamine.

In contrast, tricyclic antidepressant drugs are probably relatively ineffective in children. Meta-analysis of the efficacy of TCAs in the treatment of childhood depression has concluded that there is no evidence that they are more effective than placebo for the broad group of children with depression. They may still be useful in individual cases that are otherwise unresponsive.

Atypical antidepressants have not been adequately evaluated in childhood. There is preliminary evidence for effectiveness of nefazodone, but the use of all these classes of drug is essentially unguided by evidence and should be used, if at all, only with specialist monitoring.

Obsessive compulsive disorder

Clomipramine is the drug therapy best established by trials in children, with its serotonin reuptake inhibition being an essential part of its efficacy. In practice, the SSRIs have now largely superseded clomipramine as the first line of drug treatment, because of their greater safety. Medication treatment for childhood obsessive compulsive disorder (OCD) may need to be long-term; remissions may be prolonged if medication is combined with cognitive behaviour therapy.

Anxiety disorders

Controlled studies of TCAs for separation anxiety disorder, with or without school refusal, have produced conflicting results. Literature is starting to emerge about the use of SSRIs for children with anxiety disorders. Fluoxetine (10 to 40mg per day) may be beneficial in the treatment of anxiety disorders and selective mutism and should be considered as a second line of therapy if psychological approaches are ineffective alone. Other drugs (including benzodiazepines, buspirone and clonidine) have been advocated but do not yet have sound support from trial evidence.

Autism and other pervasive developmental disorders

Medication plays only a small role in management, which should be based largely on psychoeducational approaches and family support. SSRIs such as fluoxetine and sertraline have been used in autistic children and adults with encouraging improvements in repetitive and maladaptive behaviour in the short term. Medication should be focussed on target behaviours (such as hyperactivity) rather than on the condition as a whole. There is early trial evidence that clonidine may improve hyperactivity, irritability and oppositional behaviour in children with autism (for whom stimulants are often inappropriate because of a tendency to increase rigidity, stereotypies and induce depression and withdrawal).

Antipsychotic drugs are quite widely used in autistic spectrum disorder, in attempts to reduce repetitive and aggressive behaviours. Atypical drugs (e.g. risperidone and amisulpride) are much to be preferred in view of their side-effect profile. Even with these, however, adverse effects such as obesity (and consequent metabolic abnormalities) are sufficiently strong that long-term use should be an uncommon event, reserved for the most intractable problems, and only persisted with if there is good clinical evidence that they are indeed of value in the individual case.

Enuresis

Desmopressin (a synthetic analogue of antidiuretic hormone) is a reasonably effective and safe means of reducing the frequency of bedwetting at night, at least in the short term, and may be useful for enabling children to go on school trips or holidays from which they would otherwise be barred. Imipramine can also be useful for this purpose. However, the value of both is very small and temporary by comparison with the safe, cheap and permanently effective therapy of the enuresis alarm.

Schizophrenia

Schizophrenia is rare in children but increases rapidly in adolescence. Early onset schizophrenia is generally considered to be a variant of the adult form of schizophrenia. Outcome is particularly poor, family histories are often heavily loaded for schizophrenia, and various forms of cognitive impairment are particularly common. A multidisciplinary approach to treatment is needed and should include the family, teachers, social workers, pharmacist, paediatrician and GP. Neuroleptics are an essential component of the therapy. Acute dystonic reactions, hyperprolactinaemia and weight gain are particularly prominent adverse reactions in young people. The first choice of drug treatment is controversial; we recommend an atypical antipsychotic such as amisulpride, risperidone or olanzapine; combined with sedation if required for the control of the acute stage. In general, the algorithm for adults applies for young people too. However, the limited trial evidence suggests that clozapine is indeed effective in this group, and this is in some contrast to the rather poor outcome with other antipsychotics. The responsible psychiatrist may therefore consider an earlier recourse to clozapine, especially when (as is often the case) severe negative symptoms are persistent. Many young people with schizophrenia enter specialist residential schools or homes; it is then particularly easy for psychiatric oversight to be lost and the adolescent psychiatric team should review actively and assertively.

Psychotropic Group	Recommended dosage ranges in children & adolescents
Drugs for treatment of Hyperkinetic Disorder and ADHD	Methylphenidate 0.2–0.7mg/kg for each dose; approx 3 doses daily Dexamphetamine 0.1–0.4mg/kg for each dose; approx 3 doses daily Tricyclics e.g. imipramine 1–2mg/kg/day, clonidine 3–4mcg/kg/day
Antipsychotics in schizophrenia	Amisulpride 100–400mg/day Risperidone 2—4mg/day Olanzapine 2.5—15mg/day Quetiapine 100–400mg/day Clozapine : start with 12.5mg/day and increase up to a maximum of 500mg daily
Antipsychotics for aggression and hyperactivity	Risperidone 0.25–2.0mg daily Amisulpride 50–300mg daily Haloperidol* 0.02—0.08mg/kg/day*
Antidepressants	Fluoxetine 10—20mg/day Paroxetine 10—40mg/day Sertraline 25—100mg/day
Drugs for treatment of nocturnal enuresis	Desmopressin 20—40mcg nocte intranasally Imipramine 0.5—1.0mg/kg

*(Dystonia/dyskinesias very common in children; consider making procyclidine available to family)

Further reading

Taylor E, Sergeant J, Doepfner M, *et al.* (1998) Clinical guidelines for hyperkinetic disorder. *Eur Child Adolescent Psychiatry*, 7, 184–200.

McNicholas F, Gringras P. (2000) Guide to attention-deficit hyperactivity disorder. *Prescriber*, 5 April, 19–29.

References

Kumra S, Frazier JA, Jacobsen LK *et al.* (1996). Childhood-onset schizophrenia: a double-blind clozapine-haloperidol comparison. *Archives of General Psychiatry*, **53**, 1090–1097.

Taylor E. (1994) Physical Treatments. In Rutter M, Taylor E & Hersov L (eds) Child and Adolescent Psychiatry: Modern Approaches. Third edition. Oxford: Blackwell Scientific Publications, 880–899.

Werry JS & Aman MG. (1993) Practitioner's Guide to Psychoactive Drugs for Children and Adolescents. New York: Plenum Publishing Corporation.

The elderly

General rules

✦ The elderly have an *increased sensitivity to medications* as a result of age-related alterations in pharmacodynamics (changes in neuronal cell numbers, receptors and receptor binding) and pharmacokinetics (changes in absorption, distribution, metabolism, excretion and protein binding).

✦ *Changes in hepatic metabolism* include a decrease in the first pass effects, as well as a decrease in oxidation, reduction and hydrolysis (phase I enzymatic reactions) of drugs. Drugs metabolised by first pass effects will thus have an increased bioavailability. Lipophilic drugs will demonstrate an increased apparent volume of distribution, while this will be decreased for hydrophilic agents. Drugs with an increased volume of distribution and a decreased hepatic clearance (e.g. diazepam) and those requiring oxidation for biotransformation will thus have a greatly prolonged half-life. *Renal clearance* declines gradually with age and this may affect clearance of many drugs.

✦ As a result of this increased sensitivity, the lowest effective dosage of medications should be used: i.e. *start low, go slow, monitor effects frequently.*

✦ Always identify possible determinants of medication *noncompliance*, including social (e.g. living alone, financial situation), physical (e.g. hearing and visual loss), concomitant illness and cognitive factors.

✦ Consider the possibility of concomitant use of *over the counter (OTC) medications.*

✦ Always *consider drug toxicity* when the patient exhibits alterations in attention or cognition or any behavioural change.

✦ *Avoid polypharmacy;* the elderly are at increased risk of adverse neuropsychiatric complications from drug interactions.

✦ Highly *protein bound drugs* will have increased free plasma levels if albumin levels are reduced. This may not be reflected in routine laboratory testing of total drug concentrations only.

✦ Avoid the use of drugs which put the elderly at *risk for falls*, especially sedative-hypnotics, phenobarbitone, phenytoin.

✦ Consider the use of psychotherapy and other *nonpharmacological treatments.*

Choice of psychotropics

✦ The elderly are more sensitive to orthostatic hypotension and anticholinergic effects. *Tricyclics* should be used with caution and monoamine oxidase inhibitors (MAOIs) should be avoided. *SSRIs* and *moclobemide* may be better tolerated and have fewer cardiac effects. Of the SSRIs, the half-lives of sertraline and citalopram are prolonged in the elderly. If a tricyclic antidepressant is required, nortriptyline may be better tolerated. Amoxapine should be avoided because of its potential for causing EPS in this at risk population, as should tricyclics with a greater degree of anticholinergic activity. Trazodone and nefazodone may also be antidepressants of choice because they have fewer cardiac and anticholinergic effects. Orthostatic hypotension may need to be monitored, however. MAOIs should be avoided because of their propensity to cause orthostatic hypotension and because the dietary restrictions may be difficult to follow for some.

✦ *Electroconvulsive therapy (ECT)* is a safe and effective treatment option in this population for severe depression and for mania and may be better tolerated than pharmacotherapy in some patients.

✦ For late-onset *bipolar disorder*, lithium appears to be as effective as in early-onset cases, but long-term follow-up studies have not been done to date. Lithium toxicity may occur at levels that would be considered 'therapeutic' in younger patients. Lithium clearance is reduced in the elderly and doses may be up to 50% lower. Of AED mood stabilisers, carbamazepine has more adverse cardiac effects and needs to be monitored with ECGs in the elderly and sodium valproate may thus be preferred. The half-life of valproate may be longer in the elderly and the free fraction may also be increased.

✦ The elderly are much more susceptible to the extrapyramidal symptoms (EPS) of *antipsychotics* as well as to the orthostatic hypotension and anticholinergic effects of these agents. When indicated they should be used in much lower doses (generally one half to one third of doses in younger adults) and titrated more slowly with frequent monitoring. It is useful to monitor the elderly for Parkinsonian side effects and for tardive dyskinesia on a three monthly basis and more frequently at the onset of therapy or when making dose adjustments. Clozapine may be associated with an increased incidence of agranulocytosis in the elderly and anecdotally has not been thought as effective as in younger adults. Sertindole should not be used in the elderly because of its cardiac effects and drug interactions. Risperidone may be used in the elderly, but its half life may be increased and blood pressure should be monitored. The lesser cardiac, anticholinergic and extrapyramidal effects of sulpiride and olanzapine make these drugs of choice in this population.

✦ *Benzodiazepines* and *drugs with a high degree of anticholinergic activity* should be avoided.

✦ ECG monitoring is recommended for all elderly patients prescribed tricyclics, typical antipsychotics, and lithium. Thioridazine is particularly dangerous and should be avoided.

Psychotropic classification	Recommended drugs
Antidepressants	Moclobemide SSRIs
Antipsychotics	Olanzapine Risperidone Sulpiride
Mood stabilisers	Lithium Sodium Valproate

References

McConnell H, Duffy J. (1994) Neuropsychiatric Effects of Medical Treatment in the Elderly. In Geriatric Neuropsychiatry (J. Cummins and E. Coffey, Eds), American Psychiatric Press, Washington, D.C., U.S.A.

McConnell H, Snyder PJ. (1998) Electroencephalography in the elderly. In P. Nussbaum (Ed.), Handbook of Neuropsychology and Aging. A volume in the *Critical Issues in Neuropsychology* series (E.E. Puente & C.R. Reynolds, Eds.). Plenum Press, New York, USA.

Further reading

Breitner JCS, Welsh KA. (1995) Diagnosis and management of memory loss and cognitive disorders among elderly persons. *Psychiatric Services,* **46**, 29-35.

Coffey CE, Cummings JL. (1994). Textbook of geriatric neuropsychiatry. American Psychiatric Press, Inc., Washington D.C. , U.S.A.

Grossberg GT, Manepalli J. (1995) The older patient with psychotic symptoms. *Psychiatric Services,* **46**, 55-54.

Kennedy GJ. (1995) The geriatric syndrome of late-life depression. *Psychiatric Services,* **46**, 43.

McCall WV. (1995) Management of primary sleep disorders among elderly persons. *Psychiatric Services,* **46**, 49-55.

Norman J, Redfern SJ. (1997) Mental Health Care for Elderly People. Churchill Livingston, New York, U.S.A.

Reynolds CF. (1992) Treatment of depression in special populations. *J Clin Psychiatry,* **53** (Suppl.9), 45.

Schneider LS. (1996) Overview of generalized anxiety disorder in the elderly. *J Clin Psychiatry,* **57** (Suppl 7), 34-45.

Smith SL, Sherrill KA, Colenda CC. (1995) Assessing and treating anxiety in elderly persons. *Psychiatric Services,* **46**, 36-42.

Pregnancy and lactation

Pregnancy

Preconception

✦ For patients who are planning a pregnancy, discuss the risks and benefits of slowly withdrawing their medication; these will depend on the patient's history and the drugs being taken.

✦ Approximately 50% of pregnancies in the UK are unplanned. In view of this, when first prescribing for any woman of childbearing age, it is important to consider the 'risk' of pregnancy and the possible effects for the foetus. For example, drugs such as lithium should not be prescribed to women of childbearing age without a prior negative pregnancy test and a discussion with the patient about the risks should she conceive.

✦ Women who are taking psychotropic medication and are having problems conceiving should be given a trial off medication, if clinically appropriate. Even if there is no history of menstrual cycle irregularity and investigations such as plasma prolactin levels are all normal, there may be non-specific effects on the hypothalamic-gonadotrophin axis which may hamper conception, e.g. reduced libido.

✦ If possible avoid all drugs especially in the first trimester. For patients who are planning a pregnancy, consider withdrawing slowly their medication (depending on the nature and severity of the patient's illness). Women may be anxious about potential harm to the foetus but the risk of relapse must be considered. Individualised counselling is advised.

✦ In women maintained on agents on which there are limited data, it may be appropriate to consider switching to a recommended treatment before conception. If doubt exists as to the safety of the patient's regime in pregnancy, the clinician is advised to contact their local or national drug information service.

Pregnancy

✦ Always treat with the lowest effective dose, for the shortest time and review regularly. Progress should ideally be monitored using recognised rating scales such as BPRS, MADRS and HAM-D. This is especially important in busy clinics where patients may see more than one doctor.

✦ In most circumstances the patient who becomes pregnant while receiving effective treatment for a psychiatric disorder should remain on the treatment known to be effective for that individual.

✦ There are few data on relapse rates in pregnancy in women with a history of depression who stop their medication. Relapse may increase the risk of postpartum depression as well as cause inadequate prenatal care, poor nutrition and obstetric complications. The woman's previous psychiatric history including severity and course of illness must be taken into account when considering stopping medication. Few data exist on relapse rates in pregnant women with bipolar affective disorder who discontinue mood stabilisers.

♦ Maintaining a pregnant woman on prophylactic antipsychotic medication may be preferable to risking relapse (when higher doses of drugs may be required). Maternal relapse may also have other adverse effects on the foetus.

♦ The expected incidence of major malformations is 2 to 3% at birth with the incidence increasing to 5% by 4-5 years of age. (The incidence increases because at birth only major malformations are noted whereas by 4-5 years of age other problems such as learning difficulties and motor neurone effects are picked up.) Of these, approximately 20 to 25% will be of genetic origin, 65 to 70% will be of unknown aetiology and 1 to 3% will be caused by drugs. The expected incidence of minor anomalies is 10% and of spontaneous abortions (in clinically recognised pregnancies) 10–20%.

♦ The time of maximum teratogenic potential is approximately 17–60 days after conception, although developmental problems may still occur in the second and third trimesters.

♦ Synergy can occur among teratogenic agents. For instance, in one study it was noted that with antiepileptic medication, the incidence of major malformations with one drug was 4% whereas this increased to 23% with four AEDs. Ideally, therefore, women should be maintained on monotherapy.

♦ Try to avoid drugs that are hypotensive or anticholinergic. These effects may compound problems already seen in the patient e.g.: constipation. Sedative drugs may also worsen the fatigue experienced in pregnancy.

♦ Pharmacokinetics change during pregnancy and doses may need to be adjusted. For instance, volume of distribution increases, albumin levels decrease (and thus free levels of certain drugs e.g. phenytoin will need to be monitored), renal plasma flow increases and some liver metabolic pathways are induced resulting in lower plasma levels of some drugs. Because of this, plasma level monitoring of psychotropics should be undertaken if possible. For lithium and perhaps TCAs the dose will need to be increased. It is less certain for other drugs. See individual sections.

♦ As withdrawal effects (irritability, restlessness, continual crying, hypertonia, tachycardia and seizures) can occur in the newborn, psychotropics should be gradually withdrawn, if possible, during the three to four weeks before expected delivery. As this is not often practical, the newborn will need to be monitored closely for adverse effects.

Postpartum mood disorders

♦ Postpartum mood disorders include postpartum blues, nonpsychotic postpartum depression and puerperal psychosis (a form of affective psychosis related to bipolar disorder).

♦ Postpartum blues occurs in up to 75% of women. Symptoms such as a labile mood, tearfulness, generalised anxiety and sleep and appetite disturbance begin within a few days of delivery and typically remit by the tenth postpartum day. Drug treatment is not necessary.

◆ Postpartum depression occurs in 10 to 15% of women after childbirth and symptoms are similar to a nonpuerperal depression. Supportive counselling may be all that is required in most cases but approximately one-quarter of postpartum depressions will require treatment.

◆ Postpartum depression typically begins in the first two to six weeks after delivery but may occur later on. The Edinburgh Postnatal Depression Scale (EPDS) can be used to screen for the disorder.

◆ Postpartum depression occurs in 25% to 50% of women with a previous episode of postpartum depression and in 30% of women with a previous history of major depression. Sub-clinical depressive or anxiety symptoms during pregnancy can also increase the risk, as may social factors such as marital problems, poor support, adverse life events and social problems.

◆ Prophylactic antidepressant treatment has been shown to reduce relapse rates if given immediately after delivery. If postpartum depression does occur, women should be treated as if they have a nonpuerperal depressive illness and be given an adequate dose of antidepressant (e.g. 150mg amitriptyline) for an adequate period i.e. six months. Antidepressants that have been investigated in postpartum depression include sertraline, venlafaxine, fluoxetine as well as oestrogen and progesterone. Antidepressant choice should however be based on previous response and the adverse effect profile of the antidepressant. When deciding whether or not to treat prescribers must be aware that maternal depression may have long-term adverse effects on the psychological development of the child. This is particularly the case if the depression occurs in the first year of life.

◆ Postpartum psychosis occurs in approximately 0.1% to 0.2% (1 to 2 per 1000) of women postpartum and presents generally within the first two weeks after delivery. Symptoms include restlessness, irritability, sleep disturbance, mood lability, disorganised behaviour, delusions and hallucinations. In women with a history of postpartum psychosis the risk of developing the illness again postpartum is 30% to 50%.

◆ In women with a history of bipolar disorder, relapse rates of 30% to 50% are seen after subsequent deliveries. The maximum risk period is in the first two years after an episode of bipolar disorder. Manic symptoms are most likely to occur in the two weeks after delivery and have a more acute onset than mania occurring outside the puerperium. Because of these high relapse rates, prophylactic lithium therapy has been investigated and found to be useful if started 48 hours postpartum in women with bipolar disorder or puerperal psychosis. Oestrogen therapy is also currently being tried and preliminary results are encouraging.

◆ *For more information on mood disorders in the postpartum period see Marks and Kumar (1998) and Kendell et al. (1987).*

Drug Choice in Pregnancy

◆ There has been limited investigation of the safety of most antipsychotics and antidepressants and conflicting data published. However, there is no good evidence to support an association between these agents and an increased risk of birth defects. Drugs with which there has been the most experience are generally regarded as being the preferred option.

◆ In depression, *tricyclic antidepressants (TCAs)* are the agents of choice as there is most experience with their use. Of these there is most experience with *amitriptyline* and *imipramine*. As these drugs are sedating, cause anticholinergic effects and postural hypotension, some suggest the use of *nortriptyline* or *desipramine* (discontinued and now only available on a named-patient basis in the UK). As dose adjustments are sometimes required in pregnancy, some suggest plasma levels of antidepressants be taken before pregnancy and once each trimester. Others however recommend that they are taken before or early on in pregnancy and then if depression recurs during pregnancy, plasma levels can again be retaken and the dose adjusted according to the plasma level. For TCAs the dose may need to be increased during pregnancy with a corresponding reduction to pregravid levels by one month postpartum.

◆ In certain circumstances *SSRIs* may be appropriate but there are fewer data on their use. There are most data for *fluoxetine* which is not thought to be associated with obstetric complications or foetal malformations. Data are encouraging with *fluvoxamine, paroxetine* and *sertraline* but are still too limited to recommend their use in pregnancy.

◆ Long term effects of these agents, particularly on cognitive and language functions, are even less certain. In one study, global IQ and language development were assessed in the children of mothers taking tricyclic antidepressants (n=80) or fluoxetine (n=55) during pregnancy and in a control group (n=84). The children were evaluated between the ages of 16 and 86 months and no significant differences between the groups were found. This needs replicating.

◆ *MAOIs* should be avoided as they are known to be teratogenic in animals and there are few data available on their use in pregnancy or on pregnancy outcome.

◆ There are few data on *moclobemide, venlafaxine, nefazodone, reboxetine* and *mirtazapine* and these drugs should be avoided in pregnancy.

Of the *antipsychotics*, there are most data on *chlorpromazine* and *trifluoperazine* and so many consider these to be the agents of choice. Others think that low-potency agents (e.g. chlorpromazine) should be avoided because they have the potential to lower blood pressure and they are anticholinergic and sedating. However, this needs to be weighed up against the risk of EPS being more likely to occur with high-potency drugs that would then require treatment with anticholinergic medication. Where data does exist for antipsychotics it generally concerns their use as antiemetics where lower doses were used for short periods. Studies on the offspring of mothers treated with phenothiazines during pregnancy have failed to show an adverse effect on cognitive function in early childhood.

Depot antipsychotics are best avoided (if avoidance is not precluded by poor maternal adherence) as they may complicate drug withdrawal before the estimated delivery date. Neonatal withdrawal may also be more severe if depot preparations are used near term.

Atypical antipsychotics should generally be avoided although none has been implicated in teratogenicity. Preliminary published data for olanzapine are encouraging and experience with clozapine suggests that it is not teratogenic. Much more information is needed before either drug can be recommended.

- There are few data on the use of *anticholinergics* in pregnancy or on pregnancy outcome. *Benztropine* and *benzhexol* use in pregnancy may be associated with malformations although data are limited. *Diphenhydramine* (predominantly used in The USA as an anticholinergic) is considered to be safe by some although withdrawal effects in the newborn (tremulousness and diarrhoea) may occur. Other obvious effects include worsening constipation in the pregnant woman. Because there are few data with these agents, they should not be given routinely as prophylaxis during pregnancy. If EPS occur, some consider it best to switch to a low-potency antipsychotic that would be less likely to cause EPS. As with other psychotropic medication, gradual withdrawal three to four weeks before expected delivery should occur, if possible.

- Of the mood stabilisers, *lithium, carbamazepine* and *sodium valproate* are all teratogenic and should be avoided in the first trimester, if possible. *Lithium* use is associated with Ebstein's anomaly, which is likely to occur 10 – 20 times more frequently in the infants of women exposed to lithium in the first trimester. However, as the baseline risk for Ebstein's anomaly is 1 in 20,000, the absolute risk is only 1 in 1000 or 0.1%. This is much lower than originally thought. Nevertheless, a detailed ultrasound and foetal echocardiogram should be performed at 16 to 18 weeks to rule out cardiovascular anomalies.

The risk of abnormalities occurring must be weighed against the risk of relapse in the woman if therapy is withdrawn. Relapse rates of up to 50% have been found to occur within two to ten weeks of stopping lithium therapy in patients with bipolar disorder who were treated for an average of 30 months. The risk of relapse increases with the number of prior affective episodes, poor recovery between episodes, polytherapy and if rapid discontinuation (<2 weeks) occurs. Although some have advocated rapid discontinuation, we consider the risk of relapse to be too high in most circumstances. Relapse may also be associated with higher overall doses of medication or multiple medications. Lithium withrawal results in similar increases in relapse rates in pregnant and non-pregnant women.

Treating with the lowest effective dose of lithium may therefore be an option, as may slowly tapering the dose (over 2 to 4 weeks or longer). If lithium is to be continued, plasma levels need to be monitored closely throughout pregnancy because dose increases are invariably required. Monthly monitoring of lithium plasma levels, U & Es and TFTs should occur in the first half of the pregnancy with more frequent monitoring after that. In late pregnancy lithium levels should perhaps be monitored weekly. To lower peak plasma levels it may also be better to split the total daily dose into three or more doses a day. Dose increases are often required because, in pregnancy, the woman will have an increased volume of distribution and increased renal clearance. As volume changes at delivery and dehydration can occur it has been suggested by some that the lithium dose should be reduced by about 25% to 30% on the estimated day before delivery. As women often do not give birth on their estimated day of delivery, others have suggested hydration or dose reduction of 50% or to pre-pregnancy doses on the day of delivery. Maternal serum monitoring and adequate hydration needs to occur after delivery.

Neonatal adverse effects that have been reported include a 'floppy infant' syndrome characterised by cyanosis and hypertonicity, non-toxic goitre, hypothyroidism, nephrogenic diabetes insipidus and cardiac arrhythmias. *For more information on lithium in pregnancy see Llewellyn et al. 1998 and Yonkers et al. 1998.*

♦ Most data concerning *carbamazepine* and *sodium valproate* use in pregnancy have involved their use in women being treated for epilepsy. They are considered teratogenic and both are associated with neural tube defects with reports of the risk for carbamazepine being 0.5% to 1% and for sodium valproate, 1% to 5%. This risk may increase with the use of more than one AED and may be dose related. Dividing the total daily dose so as to lower peak plasma levels is therefore recommended. Keeping valproate levels below 70mg/L may also be beneficial.

Folic acid has been shown to help prevent neural tube defects and a dose of 4mg/day is recommended in the UK when there has been a previous child born with neural tube defects or if there is a family history. Therefore, even though there are no studies looking at the use of folic acid in women taking carbamazepine and sodium valproate, it has been suggested that folic acid be taken at a dose of 4mg/day (only 5mg is available in the UK) by women taking these drugs. Folic acid needs to be taken at least one month and perhaps for three months, before conception. RBC folate is a better indication of a patient's folate levels than is serum folate. Folic acid must then be continued for a further three months after conception. Women who are considering becoming pregnant or, as most pregnancies are unplanned, perhaps all women of child-bearing age who are taking carbamazepine or sodium valproate should therefore be taking 4mg of folic acid daily. Women who are not taking carbamazepine or sodium valproate and who are of child-bearing age need only take 400mcg of folic acid daily. In women who become pregnant on sodium valproate or carbamazepine, a high resolution ultrasound scan should be carried out at 18 weeks gestation. Maternal serum alpha-fetoprotein (AFP) levels should also be taken.

Minor anomalies have also been reported, including craniofacial abnormalities – a broad, flat nasal bridge, elongated upper lip, rotated ears and fingernail hypoplasia. With increasing age, these features appear to be less prominent. In one study, IQ was not found to be adversely affected in infants exposed to carbamazepine in utero at five-year follow-up.

To prevent neonatal haemorrhage, vitamin K (10mg/day) should be administered in the last month of gestation to mothers taking enzyme inducing agents (e.g. carbamazepine, phenytoin, phenobarbitone). Neonates at birth should be given 1mg of Vitamin K.

♦ *Gabapentin* and *lamotrigine* are being increasingly used as mood stabilisers. There are however even fewer data relating to their use in pregnancy. Lamotrigine has not been found to be teratogenic in animal studies.

♦ There are conflicting data concerning an association between *benzodiazepines* and congenital malformations although there have been suggestions of a benzodiazepine embryopathy and an association with an increased risk of facial clefts. As with all drugs, the use of benzodiazepines should be avoided, particularly in the 1st trimester. If this has not been possible it may be prudent to perform a level 2 ultrasonography to rule out visible forms of facial cleft, although only severe forms may be visualised. Prolonged use of the drugs has resulted in symptoms of neonatal withdrawal and the use of high doses close to delivery has been associated with a characteristic 'floppy infant syndrome' which includes symptoms such as hypotonia, respiratory embarrassment, hypothermia and difficulty in suckling. If a benzodiazepine is considered to be essential it should be given on a short-term basis at the minimum effective dose. There is most information for *diazepam*, *lorazepam* and *chlordiazepoxide*.

◆   *ECT* is not thought to be teratogenic in pregnancy, based on a limited number of case reports; foetal monitoring is required.

◆   If a simple hypnotic is required, *promethazine* may be safe and appropriate.

Psychotropic Group	Recommended Drugs*
Antidepressants	Nortriptyline
	Amitriptyline
	Imipramine
	Fluoxetine
Antipsychotics	Trifluoperazine
	Chlorpromazine
	? Haloperidol
Sedatives	Promethazine
Mood stabilisers	Lithium, carbamazepine and sodium valproate <u>are best avoided</u> during the first trimester
	Folic acid 4mg (5mg) should be given to all women of child-bearing age on carbamazepine and sodium valproate

There are too few data to make firm recommendations for safe drug use in pregnancy. However, the cited recommendations represent the drugs for which there is the most information available.

Lactation

General notes

◆ Research data are limited and largely inconclusive:

    ◇ Very few systematic studies have been performed.

    ◇ Evaluation is usually limited to immediate effects on the nursing infant with almost nothing known about longer-term effects.

◆ All psychotropics can be assumed to pass into breast milk, but usually milk concentration is relatively low and infant exposure slight. Nevertheless, infant adverse effects can occur.

◆ **Avoid** breastfeeding if:

Mother is taking:
    ◇ MAOIs
    ◇ Lithium
    ◇ Clozapine

Infant has evidence of:
    ◇ Renal impairment
    ◇ Hepatic impairment
    ◇ Cardiac problems
    ◇ Neurological problems

◆ If breastfeeding while taking psychotropics, avoid feeding infant when milk drug levels peak.

Time to peak (after mother's ingestion) is known for the following:

◇	Imipramine	1 hour
◇	Amitriptyline	1.5 hours
◇	Moclobemide	<3 hours
◇	Sertraline	7–10 hours
◇	Chlorpromazine	2 hours
◇	Fluvoxamine	4 hours

For other drugs, suggest giving drug as a single daily dose before the infant's longest sleep period. Breastfeeding should take place immediately before this dose is given.

◆ Monitoring of the infant should include biochemical (creatinine, LFTs, etc.) and behavioural (excessive crying, sedation, irritability).

Prescribing in lactation

✦ **Continuation therapy** (mother took psychotropic during pregnancy):-

    ✧ continue with same drug given during pregnancy but note that infant exposure will be <u>reduced</u> compared with that before birth. This may lead to withdrawal effects.

    ✧ Monitor as above and refer to paediatrician for developmental evaluation.

✦ **New therapy** (mother requires *de novo* drug treatment and wants to continue breast-feeding):

    ✧ Give lowest possible dose

    ✧ Avoid polypharmacy

    ✧ Monitor as above and refer to paediatrician for developmental evaluation

    ✧ Use drug from table below

Recommendations for prescribing in breastfeeding mothers

Psychotropic group	Recommendations
Antidepressants	Tricyclics (not doxepin) e.g. imipramine nortriptyline SSRIs – fewer data but only minor infant effects reported **Avoid** all other antidepressants unless taken by the mother during pregnancy
Antipsychotics	Chlorpromazine (≤200mg/day) Haloperidol (≤ 10mg/day) Trifluoperazine (≤ 20mg/day) *Few data so close monitoring required* **Avoid** all other antipsychotics – too few data to assure safety – unless taken by mother during pregnancy
Mood stabilisers	Valproate Carbamazepine <u>Avoid</u> lithium

References

Adis International Ltd. (1995) Neuropsychotherapeutics and breast-feeding – assess the risk:benefit ratio. *Drugs & Therapy Perspectives*, **6**, 10–12.

Adis International Ltd. (1998) Postpartum psychiatric disorders: identify early and treat aggressively. *Drugs & Therapy Perspectives*, **11**, 8–10.

Adis International Ltd. (2000) With proper care, successful pregnancy likely in women with epilepsy. *Drug and Therapy Perspectives*, **15**, 5–8.

Altshuler LL, Hendrick VC. (1996) Pregnancy and psychotropic medication: changes in blood levels. *J Clin Psychopharmacol*, **16**, 78–80.

Altshuler LL, Hendrick V, Cohen LS. (1998) Course of mood and anxiety disorders during pregnancy and the postpartum period. *J Clin Psychiatry*, **59 (suppl 2)**, 29–33.

Altshuler LL, Cohen L, Szuba MP, *et al.* (1996) Pharmacologic management of psychiatric illness during pregnancy: dilemmas and guidelines. *Am J Psychiatry*, **153**, 592–606.

Arnold LM, Suckon RF, Lichtenstein PK. (2000) Fluvoxamine concentrations in breast milk and in maternal and infant sera. *J Clin Psychopharmacol*, **20**, 491–492.

Buist A. (1997) Postpartum psychiatric disorders: guidelines for management. *CNS Drugs*, **8**, 113–123.

Chaudron LH, Jefferson JW. (2000) Mood stabilizers during breastfeeding: a review. *J Clin Psychiatry*, **61**, 79–90.

Chisholm CA, Kuller JA. (1997) A guide to the safety of CNS-active agents during breastfeeding. *Drug Safety*, **17**, 127–142.

Cohen LS, Rosenbaum JF. (1998) Psychotropic drug use during pregnancy: weighing the risks. *J Clin Psychiatry*, **59 (suppl 2)**, 18–28.

Cooper PJ, Murray L. (1998) Postnatal depression. *BMJ*, **316**, 1884–1886.

Dwight MM, Walker EA. (1998) Depressive disorders during pregnancy and postpartum. *Current Opinion in Psychiatry*, **11**, 85–88.

Duncan DA, Taylor DM. (1995) Which antidepressants are safe to use in breast-feeding mothers? *Psych Bull*, **19**, 551–552.

Ericson A, Kallen B, Wiholm B. (1999) Delivery outcome after the use of antidepressants in early pregnancy. *Eur J Clin Pharmacol*, **55**, 503–508.

Goldstein DJ. (1995) Effects of third trimester fluoxetine exposure on the newborn. *J Clin Psychopharmacol*, **15**, 417–420.

Goldstein DJ, Corbin LA, Fung MC. (2000) Olanzapine-exposed pregnancies and lactation: early experience. *J Clin Psychopharmacol*, **20**, 399–403.

Hägg S, *et al.* (2000) Excretion of fluvoxamine into breast milk. *Br J Clin Pharmacol*, **49**, 286–288.

Howe AM, Oakes DJ, Woodman PD *et al.* (1999) Prothrombin and PIVKA–11 levels in cord blood from newborn exposed to anticonvulsants during pregnancy. *Epilepsia*, **40**, 980–984.

Iqbal MM. (1999) Effects of antidepressants during pregnancy and lactation: review. *Ann Clin Psychiatry*, **11**, 237–256.

Kaneko S, Battino D, Andermann E, *et al.* (1999) Congenital malformations due to antiepileptic drugs. *Epilepsy Res*, **33**, 145–158.

Kendell RE, Chalmers JC, Platz C. (1987) Epidemiology of puerperal psychoses. *Br J Psychiatry*, **150** 662–673.

Kulin NA, Pastuszak A, Sage SR, *et al.* (1998) Pregnancy outcome following maternal use of the new selective serotonin reuptake inhibitors: a prospective controlled multicenter study. *JAMA*, **279**, 609–610.

Lee A, Donaldson S. (1995). Drugs In Pregnancy – Psychiatric and neurological disorders: part 1. *The Pharmaceutical Journal*, **254**, 87–90.

Llewellyn A, Stowe ZN. (1998) Psychotropic medications in lactation. *J Clin Psychiatry*, **59 (suppl 2)**, 41–52.

Llewellyn AM, Stowe ZN, Nemeroff CB. (1997) Depression during pregnancy and the puerperium. *J Clin Psychiatry*, **58 (suppl 15)**, 26–32.

Loebstein R, Koren G. (1997) Pregnancy outcome and neurodevelopment of children exposed in utero to psychoactive drugs: the Motherisk Experience. *J Psychiatry Neurosci*, **22**, 192–197.

McElhatton PR. (1992) The use of phenothiazines during pregnancy and lactation. *Reprod Toxicol*, **6**, 474–490.

McElhatton PR. (1994) A review of the effects of benzodiazepine use during pregnancy and lactation. *Reprod Toxicol*, **8**, 461–475.

McElhatton PR, Garbis HM, Elefant E, *et al.* (1996) The outcome of pregnancy in 689 women exposed to therapeutics doses of antidepressants. *Reprod Toxicol*, **10**, 285–294.

McElhatton. (1999) Use of antidepressants in pregnancy and lactation. *Prescriber,* **19 April**, 101–111.

Misri S, Burgmann A, Kostaras D. (2000) Are SSRIs safe for pregnant and breastfeeding women? *Can Fam Physician,* **46**, 626–633.

Murray L, Cooper PJ. (1997) Postpartum depression and child development. *Psychol Med,* **27**, 253–260.

Nonacs R, Cohen LS. (1998) Postpartum mood disorders: diagnosis and treatment guidelines. *J Clin Psychiatry,* **59 (suppl 2)**, 34–40.

Nulman I, Rovet J, Stewart DE, *et al.* (1997) Neurodevelopment of children exposed in utero to antidepressant drugs. *N Eng J Med,* **336**, 258–262.

Piontek CM, Baab S, Peindl KS, *et al.* (2000) Serum valproate levels in 6 breastfeeding mother-infant pairs. *J Clin Psychiatry,* **61**, 170–172.

Schenker S, Yang Y, Mattiuz E, *et al.* (1999) Olanzapine transfer by human placenta. *Clin Exp Pharmacol Physiol,* **26**, 691–697.

Schmidt K, Olesen OV, Jensen PN. (2000) Citalopram and breastfeeding: serum concentration and side effects in the infant. *Biol Psychiatry,* **47**, 164–165.

Stowe ZN, Cohen LS, Hostetter A, *et al.* (2000) Paroxetine in human breast milk and nursing infants. *Am J Psychiatry,* **157**, 185–189.

Trixler M, Tenyi T. (1997) Antipsychotic use in pregnancy. *Drug Safety Concepts,* **16**, 403–410.

Viguera AC, Nonacs R, Cohen LS, *et al.* (2000) Risk of recurrence of bipolar disorder in pregnant and nonpregnant women after discontinuing lithium. *Am J Psychiatry,* **157**, 179–184.

Warner JP. (2000) Evidence-based psychopharmacology 3. Assessing evidence of harm: what are the teratogenic effects of lithium carbonate? *J Psychopharmacol,* **14**, 77–80.

Weinberg MK, Tronick EZ. (1998) The impact of maternal psychiatric illness on infant development. *J Clin Psychiatry,* **59 (suppl 2)**, 53–61.

Yonkers KA, Little BB, March D. (1998) Lithium during pregnancy: drug effects and their therapeutic implications. *CNS Drugs,* **9**, 261–269.

Yoshida K, Kumar R. (1996) Breast feeding and psychotropic drugs. *Int Rev Psychiatry,* **8**, 117–124.

Yoshida K, Smith B, Kumar R. (1999) Psychotropic drugs in mothers' milk: a comprehensive review of assay methods, pharmacokinetics and of safety of breast-feeding. *J Psychopharmacol,* **13**, 76–92.

Medical co-morbidity

Cardiovascular disease

General principles:

✦ Thorough physical history and examination are fundamental to all good medical and pharmacological management.

✦ Polypharmacy with psychotropic drugs should ideally be avoided at all times, but particularly in the presence of cardiac disease.

✦ Beware of interactions with drugs producing changes in cardiac rate and in electrolyte balance.

✦ Abnormal QTc is variously defined as being >450ms, >500ms and >520ms. Prolonged QT interval may lead to torsade de pointes, which is sometimes fatal. It is not clear whether or not there is a threshold of QT prolongation which predisposes to torsades or whether the risk increases proportionally as QT prolongation increases.

✦ The elderly are at higher risk of virtually all common cardiac pathologies.

✦ Some drugs are specifically contraindicated and should be avoided e.g. pimozide. Sertindole has recently been withdrawn, except for use on a named-patient basis because of its cardiac effects and reports of sudden death – its use in cardiac patients should be considered an absolute contraindication.

✦ Avoid rapid escalation of drug doses in established cardiac disease.

Where cardiovascular disease is established, the need for starting a psychotropic drug should be reviewed in light of cardiac medications already prescribed. However, the incidence of some psychiatric illness is increased in the context of cardiac disease. For example, myocardial infarction (MI) is associated with an increased incidence of depressive illness; this in turn adversely affects the mortality post MI and should therefore be actively treated.

Specific clinical situations:

Myocardial infarction

✦ Avoid all antidepressants if possible for two months after MI. If required (see above) use SSRIs (except fluvoxamine and citalopram, which may be more cardiotoxic in overdose) or mianserin. Avoid tricyclics. If a sedative antidepressant is required, use nefazodone (beware hypotension). See page 70 for more detailed information.

✦ Avoid high dose antipsychotics. In addition to orthostatic hypotension and tachycardia, most antipsychotics have direct cardiac muscle depressant effects. This toxicity is most common with high dosing and in damaged cardiac muscle post MI. Generally, phenothiazines are more hypotensive than butyrophenones. Avoid pimozide in a patient with any cardiac abnormality in the history. Clozapine should be started slowly and with caution less than a year post MI or in cardiac disease. Olanzapine may be a safe alternative in the acute post MI, as it only rarely causes hypotension.

Heart failure

+ This may be acute or chronic. If chronic and stable, avoid drugs known to alter cardiac function, e.g. beta- blockers. Be cautious with those producing orthostatic hypotension e.g. clozapine, risperidone and quetiapine or tricyclics, nefazodone, trazodone and possibly venlafaxine. Drugs producing fluid retention, such as carbamazepine, should also be avoided or used with caution. Venlafaxine can of course cause hypertension which may be deleterious in cardiac failure.

+ If acute, the cause of the heart failure will determine which drugs are safe to use. Some hypotensive effects of psychotropics may be beneficial, especially in the context of hypertensive, high output failure. If the myocardium is unstable, it may be necessary for cardiotoxic psychotropic medication to be discontinued or avoided until the heart is stabilised.

+ Use great caution with lithium and changes in diuretic therapy.

Angina

+ Avoid drugs causing orthostatic hypotension. This may exacerbate angina by producing rebound tachycardia.

+ Phenothiazines, clozapine and risperidone amongst others can all cause tachycardia and should be used with caution.

+ Most antidepressants are thought to be safe in angina, but trazodone, nefazodone and tricyclics should usually be avoided.

Hypertension

+ Psychotropic drugs may interact with prescribed antihypertensive medication in a beneficial or dangerous manner. Orthostatic effects of psychotropic medication should be monitored closely. Patients should be monitored initially if choosing drugs with known hypotensive effects. Choice of treatment should take into account the duration of the hypertension and the state of the myocardium.

+ Sometimes the lower doses of tricyclics and antipsychotics can produce rebound hypertensive pressor responses on initiation of treatment. Avoid pimozide. Note also some dangerous interactions between some antidepressants and archaic antihypertensives (adrenergic neurone blockers).

✦   Note the possible occurrence of hypertension with clozapine and high dose venlafaxine.

Arrhythmias

For depression, SSRIs are the drugs of first choice. Note that fluvoxamine has a weak association with cardiac arrhythmias. In clinical use, citalopram appears not to affect cardiac rhythm. (See page 70.)

In psychosis, use sulpiride, olanzapine or amisulpride but avoid phenothiazines (especially thioridazine), butyrophenones and especially pimozide. Sertindole is an absolute contraindication in cardiac arrhythmias. Ziprasidone has a small effect on QTc and should be avoided.

For treatment of comorbid anxiety, it is important to differentiate between cardiac arrhythmias and panic disorder; 24 hour halter monitoring may be useful if the diagnosis is in doubt.

Notes on some specific drugs:

Lithium is contraindicated in cardiac failure and in sick sinus syndrome. Lithium commonly causes flattening of T-waves and T-wave inversion. Widening of the QRS complex has also been reported. In healthy patients a baseline ECG with yearly follow-up is desirable, although the T-wave changes are felt to be benign and often disappear with continued therapy. In patients with cardiac disease closer monitoring may be indicated. It should be used with caution in patients with pre-existing conduction abnormalities. The usual precautions and care should be exercised when prescribing with other drugs. Note the important interaction with diuretics.

Benzodiazepines are generally safe, but should be avoided in pulmonary insufficiency and acute or chronic pulmonary failure, which may be more common in heart disease. Avoid chlormethiazole in pulmonary insufficiency.

Disulfuram is contraindicated in cardiac failure, hypertensive heart disease and can produce cardiac arrest in an antabuse reaction. Best avoided.

Lofexidine should be used with caution post MI and in cardiac disease.

References

1. Rasmussen SL, Overo KF, Tanghoj P. (1999) Cardiac safety of citalopram: prospective trials and retrospective analyses. *J Clin Psychopharmacol*, **19(5)**, 407–415.
2. Reznik I, Rosen Y, Rosen B. (1999) An acute ischaemic event associated with the use of venlafaxine: a case report and proposed pathophysiological mechanisms. *J Psychopharmacol*, **13(2)**, 193–195.
3. Reilly JG, Ayis SA, Ferrier IN, *et al.* (2000) QTc-interval abnormalities and psychotropic drug therapy in psychiatric patients. *Lancet*, **355**, 1048–1052.
4. Roose SP, Spatz E. (1999) Treatment of depression in patients with heart disease (Review) *J Clin Psychiatry*, **60 (suppl 20)**, 34–37.
5. Roose SP, Spatz E. (1999) Treating depression in patients with ischaemic heart disease: which agents are best to use and avoid? *Drug Safety*, **20(5)**, 459–465.
6. Seiner SJ, Mallaya G. (1999) Treating depression in patients with cardiovascular disease (Review) *Harvard Review of Psychiatry*, **7(2)**, 85–93.
7. Welch R, Chue P. (2000) Antipsychotic agents and QT changes. *J Psychiatry Neurosci*, **25**, 154–160.

Hepatic impairment

General rules

♦ The severity of liver disease, rather than its aetiology, relates more directly to the impairment of drug metabolism. The risk of drug toxicity thus increases with the severity of the disease and in fulminant hepatic failure, drugs must be used with great care. In cholestasis, however, drug toxicity tends to be less of a problem.

♦ Clinical signs of hepatic impairment include: jaundice, ascites, encephalopathy, hypoalbuminaemia and a prolonged prothrombin time.

♦ Liver function tests are not strictly quantitative and do not correlate well with impairment of drug metabolism. It is therefore impossible to predict to what extent a drug's metabolism will be affected. In general, however, the more abnormal the liver function tests, the more severe the liver impairment and the lower the starting dose of psychotropic that should be used.

♦ Portal-systemic shunting, which may be associated with oesophageal varices, ascites or hepatic encephalopathy, allows increased systemic availability of drugs. This is important for drugs with a high (>50%) first-pass clearance by the liver and thus they should be prescribed at lower doses.

♦ Patients with liver disease may be more sensitive to type A (predictable) adverse effects of drugs even at 'therapeutic levels'.

♦ In severe liver disease, sedative drugs and drugs which cause constipation may adversely affect cerebral function and may precipitate or mask hepatic encephalopathy. Over half of patients with cirrhosis demonstrate subclinical encephalopathy on neuropsychological or neurophysiological testing, despite having no overt neuropsychiatric symptoms.

♦ In even moderate liver disease renal function may be affected. Lower doses of renally cleared drugs may therefore be required.

♦ All psychotropics should be started at a low dose and dose adjustments should be made slowly. The total dose of psychotropic should generally be lower than that considered normal.

Psychotropics

♦ There are few clinical studies on the use of psychotropics in liver disease.

♦ Most psychotropics are extensively metabolised by the liver. Therefore in liver disease psychotropic plasma levels will be increased. *Amisulpride, sulpiride, lithium* and *gabapentin* undergo no or minimal hepatic metabolism.

♦ Drugs which are highly protein bound - *TCAs, SSRIs (*except *citalopram), nefazodone, reboxetine, trazodone* and antipsychotics (except *amisulpride* and *sulpiride*) - may have increased free plasma levels. Changes such as these will not show up in measured (total) plasma levels.

- Drugs with a high first-pass clearance by the liver – e.g. *imipramine, amitriptyline, desipramine, doxepin, haloperidol* – should be started at lower doses than usual.

- *Phenothiazines* (especially *chlorpromazine)* and the irreversible *MAOIs* are hepatotoxic and should be avoided.

- If a psychotropic is added, liver function tests must be monitored weekly. If any individual parameter rises 2-3 times above baseline, withdrawal of the drug would be necessary.

Antidepressants

- With respect to the antidepressants, there is perhaps most safe clinical use with imipramine and paroxetine. *Lofepramine* is contraindicated and the more sedative TCAs such as *amitriptyline* and *dothiepin* are best avoided.

- There is less clinical experience with the newer antidepressants in liver disease, although it has been suggested that in depressed patients with a history of alcohol abuse the non-sedating SSRIs would appear preferable to TCAs. There have been published studies with *fluoxetine, paroxetine, sertraline, moclobemide* and *nefazodone* in patients with cirrhosis. The drugs' half-lives were increased and clearance reduced and so lower doses should be employed in clinically significant liver disease.

- Pharmacokinetic studies have shown that liver disorders slow the metabolism of *fluoxetine* and its active metabolite, norfluoxetine. The mean elimination half-lives in subjects with cirrhosis are 8 and 12 days respectively for fluoxetine and norfluoxetine compared with 2 to 3 and 7 to 9 days, respectively in normal patients. In well-compensated cirrhotic patients, the dose of fluoxetine should be reduced by at least 50%. In more severe liver disease, a greater reduction would be needed.

- In a single-dose study, pharmacokinetic data for *paroxetine* in patients with liver disease were similar to healthy volunteers and for this reason it has been suggested to be the SSRI of first choice. Higher plasma concentrations and reduced elimination have been seen in a 14 day multiple dose study and so it is recommended that doses at the lower end of the dose range should be used.

- The elimination half-life of *sertraline* is significantly prolonged and, as it is contraindicated in liver disease by the manufacturers and, it should be avoided.

- For *fluvoxamine* the manufacturers recommend that in patients with hepatic insufficiency, treatment should begin with a low dose (50mg a day) and the patient carefully monitored. Rarely, treatment with fluvoxamine has been associated with an increase in hepatic enzymes, usually accompanied by symptoms. The drug should be withdrawn in such cases.

- Serum concentrations of *citalopram* were measured in a group of patients with reduced hepatic dysfunction following administration of a single 20mg oral dose. Systemic clearance of citalopram was lower and the elimination half-life of the drug was longer in these patients compared with healthy volunteers with normal liver function. The manufacturer recommend that the dose of citalopram be restricted to the lower end of the dosage range.

- For *moclobemide*, the dose should be reduced by one-half to two-thirds.

- Patients with liver disease may be exposed to higher concentrations of *nefazodone* and its metabolites and so a lower daily dose should be used. Nefazodone has been associated with liver failure in three cases.

- *Reboxetine* undergoes extensive hepatic metabolism and thus the dose should be started at 2mg twice daily and increased according to efficacy and tolerability.

- Data on file for *venlafaxine* suggest that in mild liver disease (PT 14 secs) no dose reduction is required while in moderate liver impairment (PT 14-18 secs), venlafaxine's dose should be reduced by 50% which can be given once a day. There are too few data to support its use in severe liver disease.

Antipsychotics

- *Haloperidol* is often considered the antipsychotic of choice in liver disease or if there has been a history of drug-induced hepatotoxicity.

- *Sulpiride* may also be an appropriate choice. Only 5% of the drug is metabolised by the liver, although there have been occasional reports of liver toxicity.

- Few problems have been reported with *flupenthixol* and *zuclopenthixol* and so they may also be options.

- As *amisulpride* is predominately renally excreted, a dose reduction is not necessary. On theoretical grounds it may therefore be an appropriate choice in hepatic impairment but we await more data before it can be recommended.

- Lower doses of *clozapine* are required and plasma levels should be obtained, as there is some evidence that these relate to efficacy and adverse effects. A plasma level of 350mg/L should be aimed for. (Note that clozapine has caused fatal cases of hepatotoxicity.)

- Doses of up to 7.5mg of *olanzapine* have been administered safely to subjects with hepatic dysfunction. Somnolence, dizziness and hypotension were the most common adverse events in these patients. However, increased hepatic transaminase levels have been reported, which may complicate monitoring.

- The oral clearance of *quetiapine* is reduced by approximately 25% in patients with hepatic impairment. Quetiapine is extensively metabolised by the liver and should be used with caution in those with known liver impairment. The manufacturer recommends a lower starting dose of 25mg a day and increased by 25–50mg a day to an effective dose.

+ Single dose studies indicate that *risperidone* is cleared normally in patients with hepatic insufficiency and the elimination half-life of the antipsychotic fraction (risperidone and 9-hydroxy-risperidone) is unaffected. The unbound fraction of risperidone is, however, increased and this may lead to a more pronounced pharmacological effect. Risperidone should be started at 0.5mg bd and increased to a maximum of 4mg a day.

+ *Sertindole* is contraindicated in severe liver disease.

+ *Zotepine* should be prescribed with caution in patients with hepatic impairment. The dose should be started at 25mg twice daily and increased gradually according to efficacy and tolerability to a maximum of 75mg twice daily. LFTs should be monitored weekly for at least the first three months.

+ In a multiple-dose study, 40mg of *ziprasidone* was given daily to hepatically impaired subjects for 4 days. In those with mild to moderate hepatic impairment, the pharmacokinetics of ziprasidone were not altered significantly and therefore dose adjustment may not be necessary.

Mood stabilisers

+ *Valproate* has been associated with liver toxicity and so is contraindicated in active liver disease and in patients with a family history of severe hepatic dysfunction.

+ *Carbamazepine* must also be used with caution in hepatic disease.

+ *Lamotrigine* is contraindicated when there is significant hepatic impairment.

+ *Lithium* and perhaps *gabapentin* are thus the mood stabilisers of choice in liver disease.

Anxiolytics

+ If an anxiolytic is required, a short-acting *benzodiazepine* at a low dose is recommended.

+ If chlormethiazole is required, it should be started at one-third the standard dose. Chlormethiazole may be useful in the severely agitated patient who may be aggressive, but note that, unlike with benzodiazepines, its effect cannot be pharmacologically reversed.

+ The half-life of buspirone in patients with hepatic impairment is twice that in healthy individuals. The manufacturers recommend that buspirone should not be used in patients with severe hepatic disease.

+ It must be remembered that sedative drugs can precipitate hepatic encephalopathy or coma in patients with liver disease and so these drugs should be used cautiously.

Psychotropic classification	Recommended drugs
Antidepressants	Paroxetine (low dose) Imipramine [10mg tds (od in the elderly) for 2 weeks, then increase by 10mg each week until a therapeutic effect is seen]
Antipsychotics	Haloperidol (low dose) Sulpiride
Mood stabilisers	Lithium ?Gabapentin*
Anxiolytics	Lorazepam Oxazepam (Use low dose)

*Limited data for use as a mood stabiliser. It is not licensed for this use.

References

Aranda-Michel J, Koehler A, Bejarano PA, *et al.* (1999) Nefazodone-induced liver failure: report of three cases. *Ann Int Med*, **130**, 285–288.

Bergstrom RF, Beasley CM, Levy NB. (1993) The effects of renal and hepatic disease on the pharmacokinetics, renal tolerance, and the risk-benefit profile of fluoxetine. *Int Clin Psychopharmacol*, **8**, 261–266.

Daly MJ. Choice of neuroleptic in liver disease. *St James's Drug Information Centre* (letter 1996).

Daly MJ. Choice of antidepressant in liver disease. *St James's Drug Information Centre* (letter 1997).

Davis M. (1991) Hepatotoxicity of antidepressants. *Int Clin Psychopharmacol*, **6**, 97–103.

DeVane CL, Pollock BG. (1999) Pharmacokinetic considerations of antidepressant use in the elderly. *J Clin Psych*, **60(suppl 20)**, 38–44.

Dostert P, Benedetti MS, Poggesi I. (1997) Review of the pharmacokinetics and metabolism of reboxetine, a selective noradrenaline reuptake inhibitor. *Eur Neuropsychopharmacolgy*, **7 (suppl 1)**, S23–S35.

Everson G, Lasseter KC, Anderson KE, *et al.* (2000) The pharmacokinetics of ziprasidone in subjects with normal and impaired hepatic function. *Br J Clin Pharmacol*, **49 (suppl 1)**, 21S–26S.

Finlayson NDC. (1994) Drugs and the liver. *Medicine International*, 455–459.

Hale AS. New Antidepressants: use in high-risk patients. *J Clin Psychiatry*, **54**, 61–73.

Joffe P, Larsen FS, Pedersen V, *et al.* (1998) Single-dose pharmacokinetics of citalopram in patients with moderate renal insufficiency or hepatic cirrhosis compared with healthy subjects. *Eur J Clin Pharmacol*, **54**, 237–242.

Mahmood I, Sahajwalla C. (1999) Clinical pharmacokinetics and pharmacodynamics of buspirone, an anxiolytic drug. *Clin Pharmacokin*, **36(4)**, 277–287.

Morgan DJ, McLean AJ. (1995) Clinical pharmacokinetic and pharmacodynamic considerations in patients with liver disease. *Clinical Pharmacokinetics*, **29**, 370–391.

Schenker S, Bergstrom R, Wolen RL, *et al.* (1988) Fluoxetine disposition and elimination in cirrhosis. *Clin Pharmacol Ther*, **44**, 353–359.

Selim K, Kaplowitz N. (1999) Hepatotoxicity of psychotropic drugs, *Hepatology*, **29(5)**, 1347–1351.

Shin JG, Soukhov N, Flockhart DA. (1999) Effect of anipsychotic drugs on cytochrome P-450 (CYP) isoforms in vitro: preferential inhibition of CYP2D6. *Drug Metab Dispos*, **27(9)**, 1078–1084.

Snoeck E, Van Peer A, Sack M, *et al.* (1995) Influence of age, renal and liver impairment on the pharmacokinetics of risperidone in man. *Psychopharmacology*, **122**, 223–229.

Wanke LA, Silbernagel RL. (2000) Drug Consults: Antidepressant use in chronic liver disease, *Micromedex Inc.*, **90**, 1–4.

Whitwoth AB, Liensberger D, Fleischhacker WW. (1999) Transient increase of liver enzymes induced by risperidone: two case reports (letter). *J Clin Psychopharmacol*, **19(5)**, 475–476.

Renal impairment

General rules

Assessment of renal function is normally made by calculating the creatinine clearance (CrCl). The CrCl is predicted using a single measurement of serum creatinine and formulae such as that of Cockroft and Gault. The formula gives a good estimate of the glomerular filtration rate (GFR).

$$CrCl = \frac{y\,(140 - age) \times IBW}{serum\ creatinine}$$

CrCl = ml/min

y = 1.04 (females) or 1.23 (males)

IBW = kg

= 50 kg + 2.3 kg per inch over 5 foot (males)

= 45.5 kg + 2.3 kg per inch over 5 foot (females)

serum creatinine = mmol/l

This equation assumes that renal function is stable. The accuracy of the test is poor in patients with a GFR < 20ml/min, in debilitated patients and in overweight patients (use IBW).

Renal impairment is divided into three grades:

Grade	GFR	Serum Creatinine
Mild	20–50ml/min	120–200mmol/l
Moderate	10–20ml/min	200–400mmol/l
Severe	< 10ml/min	> 400mmol/l

✦ The extent of accumulation of drugs given to patients with renal impairment depends on the degree of renal dysfunction and the dose. Consequently, before an appropriate drug or dose schedule can be chosen the severity of renal impairment must be assessed.

✦ Renal function declines with age. Because many of the elderly will have reduced body mass, their GFR will be less than 50ml/min even though their serum creatinine may not be raised. It may therefore be best to assume at least mild renal impairment in the elderly.

✦ Renal impairment is an important consideration when drugs are primarily cleared by the kidney or when metabolites are pharmacologically active or toxic and are dependent on the kidney for elimination.

✦ All antidepressants and antipsychotics (with the exception of amisulpride and sulpiride) are predominatly metabolised by the liver. Generally only small amounts are excreted unchanged in the urine. The drugs may have active metabolites that are excreted renally.

✦ All psychotropics should be started at a low dose and dose adjustments should be made according to tolerability and efficacy. The drug may need to be given in divided doses. Plasma levels may be useful.

◆ Adverse effects such as postural hypotension and confusion may be more frequent in patients with renal disease. This may be because of fluid volume deficits, dialysis, autonomic insufficiency, concomitant anti-hypertensive medication or metabolic cerebral impairment. Excessive sedation can also occur frequently in patients with renal failure.

◆ Psychotropics with anticholinergic activity may cause urinary retention and interfere with precise urine measurements. The aliphatic and piperidine phenothiazines, *chlorpromazine* and *thioridazine*, and the tricyclic antidepressants, *amitriptyline* and *imipramine*, are more likely to cause these problems.

◆ There is little information about the dialysability of antipsychotics. Because they are lipid soluble, have large volumes of distribution and are highly protein bound, most would not expect to be cleared by dialysis. This is also true for the antidepressants.

Antidepressants

◆ The metabolites of *tricyclic antidepressants* are excreted by the kidneys and accumulation may occur causing an increase in adverse effects e.g. hypotension, sedation, and anticholinergic effects. Tricyclics should be started at a low dose and increased slowly according to tolerability and efficacy and the dose should be divided. Up to 50% of the dose of lofepramine is excreted unchanged by the kidneys and is best avoided in severe renal failure, although low doses have been used by patients on dialysis.

◆ Approximately 12% of *citalopram* is excreted unchanged in the urine and 20% is excreted as metabolites, some of which are pharmacologically active. There are no data on the use of citalopram in moderate to severe renal failure (ie. CrCl < 20ml/min). Dose adjustment is not considered necessary in mild renal failure.

◆ In a multiple dose study, 20mg of *fluoxetine* was given daily for more than 60 days to depressed patients with normal renal function and to renally-impaired, depressed patients who required haemodialysis. Steady state concentrations of fluoxetine in the dialysis patients were almost twice that of those with normal renal function. In mild to moderate renal failure, fluoxetine should be commenced at 10mg a day or 20mg every second day and increased only if necessary. The use of fluoxetine in severe renal failure is contraindicated by the manufacturer but in practice it is often used. Fluoxetine is not recommended for patients with a GFR of less than 10ml/min unless they are on haemodialysis.

◆ One unpublished report investigated the use of *fluvoxamine* in non-depressed patients with renal impairment. Accumulation of fluvoxamine did **not** occur with a daily dose of 100mg over 6 weeks. However, the manufacturer recommends that treatment should begin with a low dose (50mg a day) and the patient carefully monitored.

◆ In a single dose study, the mean maximum plasma concentration and half-life of *paroxetine* increased as renal function decreased. There was however wide inter-subject variability and paroxetine was well tolerated by all subjects. There have been no multiple-dose studies and there are no data on the use of paroxetine in depressed patients with a creatinine clearance less than 5ml/minute or in renal dialysis. It is highly protein bound and therefore unlikely to be removed by dialysis and additional dosing after dialysis is not necessary. Because of limited data we recommend that paroxetine be started at 10mg/day and increased only if necessary according to tolerability and efficacy. The maximum dose should be towards the lower end of the range recommended for the general population. (Liquid preparation now available.)

- In a single-dose study, 100mg of *sertraline* was administered to patients with a CrCl < 20ml/min and a control group. There were no differences in pharmacokinetic values but steady state pharmacokinetic data are not available. As sertraline has an active metabolite and as there are limited data, it should be used with caution in renal failure.

- There are limited data on the use of *MAOIs* in renal impairment but one reference suggests that dose reductions are not required for phenelzine.

- Less then 1% of *moclobemide* and approximately 6-10% of the N-oxide metabolite, which may be active, is cleared renally. In patients with different grades of renal impairment, single-dose studies showed that pharmacokinetic data do not vary amongst the group. The manufacturer recommends that dose reductions are not necessary in renal impairment.

- *Mirtazapine's* clearance is reduced in moderate to severe renal impairment and so dose adjustments may be required.

- Limited data exist on the use of *nefazodone* in renal impairment. Nefazodone is metabolised hepatically to active metabolites and with chronic administration accumulation may occur in patients with severe renal impairment. Lower doses should be used.

- The pharmacokinetics of *reboxetine* were studied in a group of 18 patients with varying degrees of renal impairment. In those with severe renal impairment, the half-life of reboxetine was increased approximately two-fold. The manufacturer recommends a starting dose of 2mg twice daily which can be increased according to patient response.

- In renal failure, *venlafaxine* clearance is reduced by up to 55%. If CrCl > 30ml/min no dose adjustment is required. If CrCl is 10–30ml/min, the daily dose should be reduced by 50% and may be given once a day if tolerated. Few data exist for patients with severe renal impairment and its use is not recommended. In haemodialysis patients, however, venlafaxine has been given at half the normal dose.

Antipsychotics

- *Chlorpromazine* has many active metabolites and renal excretion is slow. There have been reports of chlorpromazine metabolite accumulation leading to toxic psychosis and hallucinations. Because it causes sedation, postural hypotension and anticholinergic adverse effects, its use should be avoided.

- There are few data on the use of *thioridazine* in renal failure. However, as thioridazine has been associated with irreversible pigmentary retinopathy at doses greater than 600mg/day, as it causes postural hypotension and anticholinergic adverse effects and because it has active metabolites it is best to avoid its use in renal failure.

- *Trifluoperazine*, a piperazine antipsychotic, is less likely to cause sedation, postural hypotension and anticholinergic adverse effects than aliphatic and piperidine phenothiazines. Few data exist on its use in renal failure but a starting dose of 4mg/day has been suggested.

- In severe renal impairment there may be some accumulation of the metabolites of *flupenthixol* and *zuclopenthixol*. As these have little pharmacological effect a dose reduction should not be necessary.

- Few data exist on the use of *haloperidol* in renal failure. In a 48 year old patient with chronic renal failure up to 4mg of haloperidol was safely given intravenously over a thirty minute period. In an elderly patient with end-stage renal disease haloperidol was given in doses of 2–4mg/day. In a second elderly patient with moderate chronic renal failure, it was suggested that higher plasma concentrations than expected were obtained from a dose of 4mg/day. Accumulation may therefore occur. Thus, even though some have suggested no dose adjustments in renal failure others have proposed that haloperidol be initiated at low doses e.g. 1mg/day. Haloperidol is less sedative and anticholinergic and less likely to cause postural hypotension than chlorpromazine.

- *Amisulpride* is eliminated by the renal route. When GFR is between 30–60ml/min, the dose should be halved and when GFR is between 10–30ml/min, the dose should be reduced to a third. There are no data when GFR is <10ml/min and so care is needed and amisulpride should probably be avoided.

- *Clozapine* causes marked postural hypotension, sedation and anticholinergic effects. It is contraindicated in severe renal disease. In mild to moderate renal failure, the dose should be commenced at 12.5mg and then increased slowly in small increments.

- *Olanzapine* 5mg was administered to subjects with moderate or severe renal failure and to healthy subjects in an open-label, fixed-dose study. Adverse effects seen were similar between the groups, although asthenia appeared more frequently in the renally impaired subjects. Their renal status may however have predisposed them to the asthenia. Overall females experienced more adverse effects. The pharmacokinetics of olanzapine in subjects with severe renal failure compared with those subjects with normal renal function was similar. The protein binding of olanzapine was not affected by renal disease. It has there-fore been suggested that the dose of olanzapine will not change in renal failure. However, as there are few data on its use in renal failure, olanzapine should be commenced at 5mg a day and increased according to tolerability and efficacy.

- The oral clearance of *quetiapine* is reduced by approximately 25% in patients with renal impairment. The manufacturer recommends a lower starting dose of 25mg a day and increased by 25–50mg a day to an effective dose.

- Approximately 40% of the dose of 9-hydroxy-risperidone, the active metabolite of *risperi-done*, is renally excreted. In renal failure, clearance of 9-hydroxy-risperidone is reduced while its elimination half-life is increased. Clearance of the active fraction, which consists of risperidone and 9-hydroxy-risperidone, is also reduced by about 50% in patients with renal disease which may lead to a more pronounced pharmacological effect. Experience with this drug in renal failure is limited but a starting dose of 0.5mg twice a day, which may lead to a more pronounced pharmacological effect, increasing up to a maximum dose of 2mg twice a day is recommended.

- *Sertindole* may cause significant postural hypotension, but has the advantage in this popu-lation of being less sedating and less anticholinergic. Its clearance is not greatly affected by renal impairment, but experience is limited in renal failure. Sertindole is contraindi-cated with drugs that prolong the QT interval or predispose to hypokalaemia and ECG monitoring is necessary. Only named-patient use is allowed.

- As *sulpiride* is primarily excreted by the kidneys, the dose may need to be decreased or the dosage interval increased according to the level of renal impairment. The following changes have been recommended.

CrCl (ml/min)	Dose adjustment	Dose interval
30–60	70%	× 1.5
10–30	50%	× 2
<10	34%	× 3

There is no information on whether sulpiride or its conjugates are dialysable but binding to plasma protein is low (14-40%).

- In renal impairment, *zotepine* should be started at 25mg twice daily, with the dose increased gradually to a maximum of 75mg twice daily.

- In a multiple-dose study, 40mg of *ziprasidone* was given daily to 39 subjects with varying degrees of renal impairment for 7 days. In those with mild to moderate renal impairment, the pharmacokinetics of ziprasidone were not altered significantly and therefore dose adjustment may not be necessary.

Mood stabilisers/Antiepileptic drugs

- *Lithium* is contraindicated by the manufacturer in renal insufficiency. If it is considered necessary, 50–75% of the usual dose has been recommended in mild to moderate renal failure and 25–50% of the usual dose in severe renal failure. Lithium plasma levels would need to be checked frequently. Therapeutic plasma levels have been obtained when lithium has been given at a dose of 600mg three times a week after haemodialysis.

- Approximately 1–2% of unchanged *carbamazepine* and its 10–11 epoxide metabolite are excreted in the urine. There are no pharmacokinetic data in patients with renal impairment but, because there is minimal renal excretion, dose adjustments have not generally been considered necessary, although some suggest a reduction of 25% in severe renal impairment. Serum levels should, at any rate, be monitored.

- Less than 4% of *valproic acid* is excreted unchanged in the urine. It has numerous metabolites, some of which are active. It has been suggested that dose adjustments are not necessary in renal impairment but free serum valproic acid levels should be monitored as protein binding is affected and free levels may increase dramatically at times.

- If *gabapentin* is used in renal impairment, its dose must be reduced according to the following:

Creatinine clearance	Dose
60–90ml/min	400mg tds
30–60ml/min	300mg bd
15–30ml/min	300mg daily
<15ml/min	300mg alternate days

- Single-dose studies of *lamotrigine* have not shown any change in serum concentrations. Lamotrigine should, however, still be used with caution in renal failure as there may be accumulation of its glucuronide metabolite.

- Carbamazepine and *valproate* are preferred to *lithium* as mood stabilisers. They are also preferred over *lamotrigine* and *gabapentin*, having much more data relating to efficacy and safety as mood stabilisers.

- *Benzodiazepines* may accumulate in renal failure and this should be accounted for in dosing.

Psychotropic classification	Recommended drugs
Antidepressants	Tricyclic antidepressants eg. amitriptyline – initially 25mg/day and increase by 25mg/week according to tolerability and response. The daily dose should be divided initially SSRIs Most clinical experience with fluoxetine/paroxetine – start at 10mg/day
Antipsychotics	Start at low dose and increase according to tolerability and efficacy Haloperidol e.g. 1mg/day Trifluoperazine e.g. 4mg/day Flupenthixol e.g. 3mg/day Zuclopenthixol e.g. 10mg/day Some atypicals may be used – see text for details
Mood stabilisers	Carbamazepine 100mg BD and increase after 1 week to 200mg BD (Aim for a Cp > 7mg/1) Sodium Valproate 500mg MR/day (Aim for a Cp > 50mg/1)

References

Aweeka F, Jayesekara D, Horton M, *et al.* (2000) The pharmacokinetics of ziprasidone in subjects with normal and impaired renal function. *J Clin Pharmacol*, **49 (suppl 1)**, 27S–33S.

Bennett WM, Aronoff GR, Golper TA, *et al.* (1991) *Drug prescribing in renal failure.* 2nd Ed. American College of Physicians, Philadelphia.

Bergstrom RF, Beasley Jr CM, Levy NB, *et al.* (1993) The effects of renal and hepatic disease on the pharmacokinetics, renal tolerance, and risk-benefit profile of fluoxetine. *Int Clin Psychopharmacol* **8**, 261–266.

Boyd RA, Turck D, Abel RB, *et al.* (1999) Effects of age and gender on single-dose pharmacokinetics of gabapentin. *Epilepsia*, **40(4)**, 474–479.

DeVane CL, Pollock BG. (1999) Pharmacokinetic considerations of antidepressant use in the elderly. *J Clin Psychiatry*, **60 (suppl 20)**, 38–44.

Dostert P, Benedetti MS, Poggesi I. (1997) Review of the pharmacokinetics and metabolism of reboxetine, a selective noradrenaline reuptake inhibitor. *Eur Neuropsychopharmacolgy*, **7 (suppl 1)**, S23–S35.

Doyle GD, Laher M, Kelly JG, *et al.* (1989) The pharmacokinetics of paroxetine in renal impairment. *Acta Psychiatr Scan* **80**, 89–90.

Gitlin M. (1999) Lithium and the kidney : an updated review. *Drug Safety*, **20(3)**, 231–243.

Joffe P, Larsen FS, Pedersen V, *et al.* (1998) Single-dose pharmacokinetics of citalopram in patients with moderate renal insufficiency or hepatic cirrhosis compared with healthy subjects. *Eur J Clin Pharmacol*, **54**, 237–242.

Schrier RW, Gambertoglio JG, (eds). (1991). Handbook of drug therapy in liver and kidney disease. Little, Brown and Co., Boston.

Snoeck E, Van Peer A, Sack M, *et al.* (1995) Influence of age, renal and liver impairment on the pharmacokinetics of risperidone in man. *Psychopharmacol* **122**, 223–229.

Psychiatric effects of medical therapies

♦ Drug-induced psychiatric dysfunction is an important consideration in the differential diagnosis of medical patients with psychiatric co-morbidity. Such effects are common and may relate to direct or indirect CNS toxicity due to the specific agent, pharmacokinetic or pharmacodynamic interactions with psychotropics or with other medical therapies or to interactions with the patient's underlying medical or psychiatric diagnosis.

♦ Psychiatric illness often goes undiagnosed in patients with medical co-morbidity, particularly in a hospital setting. The effects of illness or of drugs may alter the presentation.

♦ The clinician must be aware of both the effects of medical therapies on psychiatric presentation as well as the effects of psychotropics on the patient's medical condition and the potential for drug interactions between the two. For example, MAOIs and moclobemide are contraindicated in phaeochromocytoma and hyperthyroidism (tranylcypramine and moclobemide) and lithium may be contraindicated in hypothyroidism and Addison's disease. In GI illness, SSRIs may exacerbate nausea while tricyclics and other anticholinergics may exacerbate constipation and their levels may be increased by concomitant use of cimetidine. In prostatic hypertrophy, tricyclics and other agents with anticholinergic properties can cause urinary retention and, in narrow angle glaucoma, they are contraindicated as they may precipitate an acute crisis. MAOIs are not recommended in the elderly, congestive heart failure, and after CVAs. Tricyclics are contraindicated in heart block and following myocardial infarction. Prescribing of psychotropics in renal disease, liver impairment, cardiac illness and in neuropsychiatric conditions is discussed in other sections of these guidelines.

♦ Drug interactions frequently exacerbate both the psychiatric symptoms and the medical condition. CNS toxicity may develop from lithium and sumatriptan in a person with migraine, for example, or from fluoxetine and selegiline in Parkinson's disease presenting with confusion. The common analgesic dextropropoxyphene frequently causes serious interactions with many drugs such as carbamazepine, increasing levels precipitously. Such interactions affecting care need not be pharmacokinetic only. Psychotropics causing postural hypotension may have additive effects with diuretics. In patients with agranulocytosis or with marrow suppression from chemotherapeutic agents, tricyclics, mianserin, carbamazepine and clozapine are all contraindicated. Drug interactions with warfarin, antiepileptic drugs, cardiac medications and psychotropics are further discussed in other sections of these guidelines.

♦ Many agents have been implicated in causing *delirium and cognitive impairment*. Of the cardiovascular medications, beta-blockers have been most implicated in producing depression, an acute confusional state, hallucinosis, sleep disruption and chronic fatigue symptoms. These risks are not, however as great as originally feared. Digoxin, quinidine, disopyramide, clonidine, methyl-dopa and others may also cause acute confusional states and/or cognitive impairment. Anticholinergics, tricyclic antidepressants, and antihistamines frequently cause delirium, particularly in the elderly. Antiparkinson agents and nonsteroidal anti-inflammatory drugs (NSAIDs) have also been implicated.

♦ *Anxiety* may be caused by stimulant use or abuse and is most common with caffeinism. Ten to 15% of patients receiving dopaminergic agents will experience anxiety as an adverse effect. Thyroxine, various cardiac drugs, theophylline and sympathomimetics may also cause anxiety. The elderly may have a paradoxical excitement with associated anxiety with benzodiazepines, barbiturates and other sedative-hypnotics. The withdrawal effects of sedative-hypnotics frequently precipitate anxiety.

- *Depression* may be caused by many agents, including propranolol, digoxin (particularly in the elderly), methyldopa, corticosteroids, NSAIDs, cimetidine, antipsychotics and others.

- *Mania and/or psychosis* have been reported with digoxin, quinidine, procainamide, disopyramide, corticosteroids, NSAIDs, antiparkinsonian agents, cimetidine and many other medical therapies. Some of the major psychiatric effects of medical therapies are listed in the following table (Modified from McConnell and Duffy, 1994).

Drug	Psychiatric effects
Antihypertensive drugs	
Clonidine	depression, mania, agitation
Propranolol	depression, mania, delirium, psychosis
Nifedipine	depression
Captopril	mania, agitation
Antiarrhythmics	
Procainamide	depression, mania, delirium, psychosis
Lignocaine	depression, delirium, psychosis
Disopyramide	delirium, psychosis
Antimicrobial agents	
Penicillins	depression, agitation, visual hallucinations
Tetracycline	depression, hallucinations
Cephalosporins	delirium, psychosis
Antimalarials	psychosis, visual hallucinations
Antiparkinson drugs	
Anticholinergics	delirium, psychosis, visual hallucinations, dementia
Amantadine	depression, agitation, delirium, psychosis, visual hallucinations
Levodopa	depression, mania, anxiety, agitation, psychosis, visual hallucinations, delirium, cognitive impairment
Antihistamines	
H1 blockers (diphenhydramine)	delirium
H2 blockers (cimetidine)	depression, mania, delirium, psychosis, visual hallucinations

Antineoplastic drugs	
Interferon	depression, agitation, delirium
Vincristine	depression
C- asparaginase	depression, delirium, psychosis
Endocrine agents	
Corticosteroids	depression, mania, psychosis, delirium
Oral contraceptives	depression
Thyroxine	anxiety, agitation, mania, psychosis, visual hallucinations
Antiepileptic drugs	
Barbiturates (phenobarbitone primidone)	hyperactivity (esp. in children), sedation, sexual dysfunction, aggression, learning deficits, cognitive impairment, depression, personality change; Positive effects: anxiolytic/hypnotic
Benzodiazepines (clonazepam, diazepam)	aggression, confusion, depression, disinhibition, irritability, cognitive impairment; Positive effects: anxiolytic/hypnotic; antimanic (clonazepam)
Carbamazepine	depression, irritability, sexual dysfunction, mania; Positive effects: antidepressant, antimanic, treatment of aggression and bipolar disorder
Clobazam	similar side effect profile to other benzodiazepines but may have lower overall incidence of cognitive and behavioural side effects; ?Anxiolytic/positive psychotropic effects
Gabapentin	sedation, ataxia, aggression and hyperactivity (children); few drug interactions; ? positive psychotropic effects
Hydantoins (phenytoin)	sedation, ataxia, dementia, affective disorder, confusion, cognitive impairment, progressive encephalopathy; Positive effects: ? antiaggressive, ?anxiolytic effects
Lamotrigine	may have additive toxicity when used with carbamazepine, ataxia, dizziness; ? positive psychotropic effects
Succinimides (ethosuximide, methsuximide)	psychosis ("alternating psychosis" – adolescents, young adults), drowsiness, insomnia, irritability, ? cognitive effects, personality change ; Positive effects: improvement in attention / concentration (likely related to seizure improvement)
Tiagabine	? depression, psychosis, ? anxiolytic effects, ? effects in tardive dyskinesia
Topiramate	sedation, confusion, cognitive dysfunction, asthenia
Valproate	progressive encephalopathy, dementia, depression, extrapyramidal effects; Positive effects: antimanic, treatment of aggression and bipolar disorder
Vigabatrin	depression, psychosis

References

Brown TM, Stoudmire A. (1998) Psychiatric side effects of prescription and over-the-counter medications: recognition and management. 1ˢᵗ Ed. American Psychiatric Press, Inc, Washington DC.

Saravay SM. (1996) Psychiatric interventions in the medically ill: outcome and effectiveness research. *Psychiatric Clinics of North America* **19**, 467–480.

Stoudemire A. (1996) New antidepressant drugs and the treatment of depression in the medically ill patient. *Psychiatric Clinics of North America* **19**, 495–513.

Neuropsychiatric conditions

I) Alcohol and substance misuse

Pharmacotherapy for alcohol withdrawal

✦ Alcohol withdrawal is associated with significant morbidity and mortality when improperly managed.

✦ All patients need general support; a proportion will need pharmacotherapy to modify the course of reversal of alcohol-induced neuroadaptation.

✦ Benzodiazepines are recognised as the treatment of choice for alcohol withdrawal. They are non-tolerant with alcohol and have anticonvulsant properties.

✦ Parenteral vitamin replacement is an important adjunctive treatment for the prophylaxis and/or treatment of Wernicke-Korsakoff syndrome and other vitamin-related neuropsychiatric conditions.

✦ The majority of patients can be detoxified in the community. However, in-patient detoxification is indicated where there is:

   A history of delirium tremens or withdrawal seizures
   A history of failed community detoxification
   Poor social support
   Cognitive impairment

The alcohol withdrawal syndrome

In alcohol-dependent drinkers, the CNS has adjusted to the constant presence of alcohol in the body. When the blood alcohol level (BAC) is suddenly lowered, the brain remains in a hyperactive and hyperexcited state causing the withdrawal syndrome.

The alcohol withdrawal syndrome is not a uniform entity. It varies significantly in clinical manifestations and severity. Symptoms can range from mild insomnia to delirium tremens (DTs).

The first symptoms and signs occur within hours of the last drink and peak within 24–48 hours. They include restlessness, tremor, sweating, anxiety, nausea, vomiting, loss of appetite and insomnia. Tachycardia and systolic hypertension are also evident. Generalised seizures occur rarely, usually within 24 hours of cessation. In delirium tremens there is confusion, disorientation, agitation, tachycardia and hypertension. Fever is common. Visual and auditory hallucinations and paranoid ideation are also seen.

In most patients symptoms of alcohol withdrawal are mild to moderate and disappear within 5–7 days after the last drink. In more severe cases (approx. 5% of cases), DTs may develop.

Risk factors for DTs and seizures

✦   Severe alcohol dependence
✦   Past experience of DTs
✦   Longstanding history of alcohol dependence with previous episodes of in-patient treatment
✦   Older age
✦   Concomitant acute illness
✦   Severe withdrawal symptoms when presenting for treatment

Alcohol withdrawal assessment

1. History (including history of previous episodes of alcohol withdrawal)
2. Physical examination
3. Time of most recent drink
4. Concomitant drug intake
5. Severity of withdrawal symptoms
6. Co-existing medical/psychiatric disorders
7. Laboratory investigations : BAC; FBC; U&E; LFTs; INR; urinary drug screen

Withdrawal scales can be helpful. They can be used as a baseline against which withdrawal severity can be measured over time. Use of these scales can minimise over- and under-dosing with benzodiazepines.

The Clinical Institute Withdrawal Assessment for Alcohol-Revised Version (CIWA-Ar) is a 10-item scale that can be used to monitor the clinical course of alcohol withdrawal. (Items 1–9 are scored from 0–7 and item 10 from 0–4; maximum possible score of 67).

1. Nausea and vomiting
2. Tremor
3. Paroxysmal sweats
4. Anxiety
5. Agitation
6. Tactile disturbances
7. Auditory disturbances
8. Visual disturbances
9. Headache and fullness in head
10. Orientation and clouding of sensorium

Severity of alcohol withdrawal	CIWA-Ar score
mild	<10
moderate	10–20
severe	20+

Chlordiazepoxide

Out-patient/Community detoxification

Mild dependence usually requires very small doses of chlordiazepoxide, or else may be managed without medication.

Moderate dependence requires a larger dose of chlordiazepoxide. A typical regime might be 10–20mg qds, reducing gradually over 5 days. Note that 5–7 days' treatment is adequate *and longer treatment is rarely helpful or necessary.*

Example:
- Day 1 .... 20mg qds
- Day 2 .... 15mg qds
- Day 3 .... 10mg qds
- Day 4 .... 5mg qds
- Day 5 .... 5mg bd

Severe dependence requires even larger doses of chlordiazepoxide and will often require specialist/in-patient treatment. Daily monitoring is advised for the first 2–3 days, especially for severe dependence (see below). This may require special arrangements over a weekend. Prescribing should not start if the patient is heavily intoxicated, and in such circumstances they should be advised to return in a sober state at an early opportunity.

In-patient protocol

The approach advocated here is to prescribe chlordiazepoxide according to a flexible regimen over the first 24 hours, with dosage titrated against the rated severity of withdrawal symptoms. This is followed by a fixed 5-day reducing regimen, based upon the dosage requirement estimated during the first 24 hours.

Occasionally (e.g. in delirium tremens) the flexible regime may need to be prolonged beyond the first 24 hours. However, rarely (if ever) is it necessary to resort to the use of other drugs, such as antipsychotics (associated with reduced seizure threshold) or intravenous chlormethiazole (associated with risk of overdose).

The intention of the flexible protocol for the first 24 hours is to titrate dosage of chlordiazepoxide against severity of alcohol withdrawal symptoms. It is necessary to avoid either under-treatment (associated with patient discomfort and a higher incidence of complications such as seizures or DTs), or over-treatment (associated with excessive sedation and risk of toxicity/interaction with alcohol consumed prior to admission).

In the in-patient setting it is possible to be more responsive, with constant monitoring of the severity of withdrawal symptoms, linked to the administered dose of chlordiazepoxide.

Prescribing

First 24 hours (day 1)

On admission, the patient should be assessed by a doctor and prescribed chlordiazepoxide. (Diazepam is used in some centres and may be used for those with a history of sensitivity to chlordiazepoxide although some metabolites are shared). Three doses of chlordiazepoxide must be specified:

First dose (stat)

This is the first dose of chlordiazepoxide which will be administered by ward staff immediately following admission, as a fixed "stat" dose. It should be estimated upon:

✦ Clinical signs and symptoms of withdrawal (see below)

✦ Breath alcohol concentration on admission and 1 hour later

The dose prescribed should usually be within the range of 5–50mg. However, if withdrawal symptoms on admission are mild, or if the breath alcohol is very high, or rising, the initial dose may be 0mg (i.e. nothing). It is the relative fall in blood alcohol concentration that determines the need for medication not the absolute figure (hence the need to take two Alcometer readings at an interval soon after admission). Caution is needed if a patient shows a high Alcometer level.

Incremental dose (range)

This is the range within which subsequent doses of chlordiazepoxide should be administered during the first 24 hours (see below). A dose of 5–40mg will cover almost all circumstances.

Maximum dose in 24 hours

This is the maximum cumulative dose which may be given during the first 24 hours. It may be estimated according to clinical judgement, but **250mg should really be adequate for most cases.** Doses above 250mg should not be prescribed without prior discussion with a Consultant or Specialist Registrar.

The cumulative chlordiazepoxide dose administered during the initial 24 hour period assessment is called the BASELINE DOSE, and this is used to calculate the subsequent reducing regime.

Days 2–5

After the initial 24-hour assessment period a standardised reducing regime is used. Chlordiazepoxide is given in divided doses, four times daily. The afternoon and evening doses can be proportionately higher in order to provide night sedation (but note that the effect of chlordiazepoxide and its metabolites is long-lived). The dose should be reduced each day by approximately 20% of the Baseline Dose, so that no chlordiazepoxide is given on day 6. **However, a longer regime may be required in the case of patients who have DTs or a history of DTs. This should be discussed with a senior registrar or consultant, and the dose tailored according to clinical need.**

Note

◇ Chlordiazepoxide should not routinely be prescribed on a PRN basis after the initial assessment is complete. Patients exhibiting significant further symptoms may have psychiatric (or other) complications and should be seen by the ward or duty doctor.

Observations and administration

After chlordiazepoxide has been prescribed as above, the first "stat" dose is given immediately. Subsequent doses during the first 24 hours are administered with a frequency and dosage which depend upon the observations of alcohol withdrawal status rated by the ward staff.

Observations

Each set of observations consist of:

✦   Applying an alcohol withdrawal scale (e.g. CIWA-Ar) and/or clinical observations

✦   Taking BP

✦   Taking pulse

✦   Alcometer (first and second observations only)

Observations should be recorded:

I)   During the admission procedure, immediately after the patient has arrived on the ward.

II)   Throughout the first 24-hours, at a frequency depending upon:
          ✦ Severity of withdrawal
          ✦ Whether or not chlordiazepoxide has been administered

III)   Twice daily from days 2–6.

If a patient is asleep (and this is not due to intoxication) they should not be woken up for observations. However, it should be recorded that they were asleep.

During the first 24 hours chlordiazepoxide should be administered when withdrawal symptoms are considered significant (usually a CIWA-Ar score of more than 15). If a patient suffers hallucinations or agitation, an increased dose should be administered, according to clinical judgement.

Alcohol withdrawal treatment interventions

Severity	Supportive care	Medical care	Pharmacotherapy for neuroadaptation reversal	Setting
mild CIWA-AR < 10	moderate to high level required	little required	little to none required – maybe symptomatic treatment only (e.g. paracetamol)	home
moderate CIWA-Ar 10–20	moderate to high level required	little required	little to none required – maybe symptomatic treatment only	home or community
severe CIWA-Ar > 20	high level required	medical monitoring	usually required – probably symptomatic and substitution treatment (e.g. chlordiazepoxide)	community or hospital
complicated CIWA-Ar > 10 plus medical problems	high level required	specialist medical care required	substitution and symptomatic treatments probably required	hospital

Example of a chlordiazepoxide regimen

		Total mg
Day 1 (first 24 hours)	40mg qds + 40mg PRN	200
Day 2	40mg qds	160
Day 3	30mg tds and 40mg nocte (or 30mg qds)	130 120
Day 4	30mg bd and 20mg bd (or 25mg qds)	100
Day 5	20mg qds	80
Day 6	20mg bd and 10mg bd	60
Day 7	10mg qds	40
Day 8	10mg tds or 10mg bd and 5mg bd	30
Day 9	10mg bd (or 5mg qds)	20
Day 10	10mg nocte	10

Vitamin supplementation

Parenteral vitamin supplements should be prescribed prophylactically for *all* in-patient detoxifications. There is considerable doubt about the usefulness of oral replacement.

Parenteral vitamin supplements should only be administered where suitable resuscitation facilities are available. The intramuscular route is usually used. Intravenous administration should be by dilution in 50–100ml normal saline and infused over 15–30 minutes. This allows immediate discontinuation should anaphylaxis occur. Anaphylaxis is extremely rare after i.m. administration and this is the preferred route in most centres.

The classical triad of ophthalmoplegia, ataxia and confusion is rarely present in Wernicke's encephalopathy and the syndrome is much more common than is widely believed. A presumptive diagnosis of Wernicke's encephalopathy should therefore be made in any patient undergoing detoxification who experiences any of the following signs:

Ataxia	Hypothermia & hypotension
Confusion	Ophthalmoplegia/nystagmus
Memory disturbance	Coma/unconsciousness

Parenteral B-complex must be admistered before glucose is administered in all patients presented with altered mental status.

Prophylactic treatment for Wernicke's encephalopathy should be:

One pair IM/IV ampoules high potency B-complex vitamins (Pabrinex) daily for 3–5 days. (Or: thiamine 200–300mg IM daily if Pabrinex unavailable)

NB. All patients should receive this regime as an absolute minimum.

Therapeutic treatment of Wernicke's encephalopathy should be:

At least two pairs IM/IV ampoules high potency B-complex vitamins daily for 2 days.

✦ No response, then discontinue treatment.

✦ If signs/symptoms respond, continue 1 pair ampoules daily for 5 days or for as long as improvement continues.

For out-patient detoxification, the options available are:

✦ No vitamin supplementation. (Not recommended.)

✦ Oral vitamin supplementation with Vitamin B Compound Strong, one tablet 3 times daily (but this is unlikely to be absorbed effectively and is therefore of little or no benefit to alcohol dependent patients).

✦ Parental supplementation, as above, in a clinical setting where appropriate resuscitation facilities are available.

Seizure prophylaxis

There is no clear consensus on seizure prophylaxis. Most clinicians prefer to use diazepam for medically assisted withdrawal in those with a previous history of seizures. Some units advocate carbamazepine loading in patients with untreated epilepsy; those with a history of more than two seizures during previous withdrawal episodes; or previous seizures despite adequate diazepam loading. Phenytoin does not prevent alcohol-withdrawal seizures and is therefore not indicated.

Those who have a seizure for the first time should be investigated to rule out an organic disease or structured lesion.

Liver disease

For individuals with impaired liver functioning, oxazepam (a short acting benzodiazepine) may be preferred to chlordiazepoxide, in order to avoid excessive build up of metabolites and over-sedation.

Hallucinations

Mild perceptual disturbances usually respond to chlordiazepoxide. However, hallucinations should be treated with oral haloperidol. Haloperidol may also be given intramuscularly or intravenously if necessary (but BP should be monitored for hypotension). Caution is needed because haloperidol can reduce seizure threshold. Have parenteral procyclidine available in case of dystonic reactions.

Symptomatic pharmacotherapy

Dehydration:
Ensure adequate fluid intake in order to maintain hydration and electrolyte balance. Dehydration can lead to cardiac arrythmia and death.

Pain: Paracetamol.

Nausea & vomiting:
Metoclopramide (Maxolon) 10mg or prochlorperazine (Stemetil) 5mg 4–6 hourly or intramuscular.

Diarrhoea:
Diphenoxylate hydrochloride and atropine (Lomotil). Loperamide-hydrochloride (Immodium).

Hepatic encephalopathy: Lactulose.

References

Claassen CA, Adinoff B. (1999) Alcohol withdrawal syndrome: guidelines for management. *CNS Drugs*, **12**, 279–291.

Duncan D, Taylor D. (1996) Chlormethiazole or chlordiazepoxide in alcohol detoxification. *Psychiatric Bulletin*, **20**, 599–601.

Mayo-smith MF. (1997) Pharmacological management of alcohol withdrawal. *JAMA*, **278**, 144–151.

Prescribing for opioid dependence

These guidelines are intended to provide information on the short-term management of patients presenting with opioid dependence. Long-term management should involve referral or contact with specialist services for advice.

Evidence of opioid dependence

Patient's self-reporting of opioid dependence must be confirmed by positive urine results for opioids, and objective signs of withdrawal or general restlessness should be present before considering to prescribe any substitute pharmacotherapy. Recent sites of injection may also be present.

Treatment aims
✦   To reduce or prevent withdrawal symptoms

✦   To stabilise drug intake and lifestyle

✦   To reduce drug related harm (particularly injecting behaviour)

✦   To help maintain contact and provide an opportunity to work with the patient

Treatment
This will depend upon:

✦   What is available

✦   Patient's previous history

✦   Patient's current drug use and circumstances

Substitute prescribing of Methadone

Methadone is a controlled drug with a high dependency potential and a low lethal dose. Prescribing should only commence if:

✦   Opioid drugs are being taken on a regular basis (typically daily)

✦   There is convincing evidence of dependence (see above)

✦   Consumption of methadone can be supervised, especially for the initial doses

Supervised daily consumption is recommended for new prescriptions, for a minimum of three months, if possible. Alternatively, instalment prescriptions for daily dispensing and collection should be used. Certainly no more than one week's supply should be dispensed at one time, except in very exceptional circumstances.

Methadone should be prescribed in the oral liquid formulation (mixture or linctus). Tablets are likely to be crushed and inappropriately injected, and therefore should not be prescribed.

Important: All patients starting a methadone treatment programme must be informed of the risks of toxicity and overdose, and the necessity for safe storage.

Dose

For patient's who are ***currently prescribed*** methadone and if ALL the criteria listed below are met, then it is safe to prescribe the same dose:

✦ Dose confirmed by prescriber

✦ Last consumption confirmed (e.g. pharmacy contacted) and is within last three days

✦ Prescriber has stopped prescribing, and current prescription is completed or cancelled to date

✦ Patient is comfortable on dose (no signs of intoxication/withdrawal)

✦ No other contraindications or cautions are present

Otherwise the following recommendations should be followed.

Starting Dose

Consideration must be given to the potential for opioid toxicity, taking into account:

✦ Patient's tolerance, which should be assessed on the history of quantity, frequency and route of administration (be aware of the likelihood of overreporting). A person's tolerance to methadone can be affected within three to four days of not using, caution must be exercised when re-instating their dose.

✦ Use of other drugs, particularly depressants e.g. alcohol and benzodiazepines.

✦ Long half-life of methadone, as cumulative toxicity may develop.

Inappropriate dosing can result in potentially fatal overdose, particularly in the first few days. Deaths have occurred following the commencement of a daily dose of 40mg methadone. It is safer to keep to a low dose that can subsequently be increased at intervals if this dose later proves to be insufficient.

Direct conversion tables for opioids and methadone should be viewed cautiously, as there are a number of factors influencing the values at any given time. It is much safer to titrate the dose against presenting withdrawal symptoms.

The initial total daily dose for most cases will be in the range of 10–40mg methadone, depending on the level of tolerance (low: 10–20mg, moderate: 25–40mg).
Starting doses greater than 30mg should be prescribed with caution, because of the risk of overdose. It is safer to use a starting dose of 10–20mg and re-assess the patient after a period of four hours. Further incremental doses of 5–10mg can be given, depending on the severity of the withdrawal symptoms. Note: onset of action should be evident within half an hour, with peak plasma levels being achieved after approximately four hours of dosing.

Heavily dependent users with high tolerance may require larger doses. A starting dose, not exceeding 30mg, can be given, followed by a second dose after a minimum interval of four hours. The second dose can be up to 30mg, depending on the persisting severity of withdrawal symptoms. Such doses should only be prescribed by experienced medical practitioners.

Severity of withdrawal after initial dose dosage	Additional
Mild	Nil
Moderate (muscle aches & pains, pupil dilation, nausea, yawning, clammy skin)	5–10mg
Severe (vomiting, profuse sweating, piloerection, tachycardia, elevated BP)	20–30mg

Stabilisation dose

✦ **First week**:
Out-patients should attend daily for the first few days to enable assessment by the prescriber and any dose titration against withdrawal symptoms. Dose increases should not exceed 5–10mg a day and 30mg a week above the initial starting dose. Note that steady state plasma levels are only achieved five days after the last dose increase.

✦ **Subsequent period**:
Subsequent increases should not exceed 10mg per week, up to a total daily dose of 60–120mg. Stabilisation is usually achieved within six weeks but may take longer.

Cautions

✦ **Intoxication.** Methadone should not be given to any patient showing signs of intoxication, especially due to alcohol or other depressant drugs e.g. benzodiazepines. Risk of fatal overdose is greatly enhanced when methadone is taken concomitantly with alcohol and other respiratory depressant drugs. Concurrent alcohol and illicit drug consumption must be borne in mind when considering subsequent prescribing of methadone.

✦ **Severe hepatic/renal dysfunction**. Metabolism of methadone may be affected and so lower doses will be required. Because of extended plasma half-life, the interval between assessments during initial dosing may need to be extended.

Overdose

In the event of methadone overdose Naloxone should be administered, if available.

Dose: by intravenous injection, 0.8–2mg repeated at intervals of 2–3 minutes to a maximum of 10mg if respiratory function does not improve.

By subcutaneous or intramuscular injection: as intravenous injection but only if intravenous route not feasible (onset of action slower).

By continuous intravenous infusion, 2mg diluted in 500ml intravenous infusion solution at a rate adjusted according to response.

Call Emergency Services

Pregnancy & breastfeeding

There is no evidence of an increase in congenital defects. It is important to prevent the patient going into a withdrawal state, since this is dangerous for both mother and foetus. Specialist advice should be obtained before prescribing, particularly with regards to management and treatment plan during pregnancy.

Methadone is considered compatible with breastfeeding, with no adverse effects to nursing infant when mother is consuming 20mg/24 hours or less.

Analgesia for Methadone prescribed patients

Non-opioid analgesics should be used in preference, e.g. paracetamol, NSAIDs.

If opioid analgesia is indicated, e.g. codeine, dihydrocodeine, MST, then this should be titrated accordingly against pain relief, with the methadone dose remaining constant to alleviate withdrawal symptoms. Avoid titrating the methadone dose to provide analgesia.

Opiate detoxification and reduction regimes

Community setting

✦ **Methadone**

Following a period of stabilisation with methadone, a contract should be negotiated between the patient and prescriber to reduce the daily methadone dose by 5–10mg weekly or fortnightly. However, this should be reviewed regularly and remain flexible to adjustments and changes in the patient's readiness for total abstinence.

✦ **Lofexidine**

Lofexidine is licensed for the management of symptoms of opioid withdrawal. It is non-opioid and therefore less liable to misuse and diversion. Its use in community detoxification is more likely to be successful for patients with an average daily heroin use of up to 1/2g (or 30mg methadone equivalent), for non-polydrug users and for those with shorter drug and treatment histories, or for those at an end stage of methadone detoxification (patients taking not more than 20mg daily).

Precautions: severe coronary insufficiency, recent MI, bradycardia, cerebrovascular disease, chronic renal failure, pregnancy and breastfeeding.

Interactions: alcohol and other CNS depressants—lofexidine may enhance the effects. Tricyclic antidepressants—concomitant use may reduce the efficacy of lofexidine.

Side effects: drowsiness, dryness of mouth, throat and nose, hypotension, bradycardia and rebound hypertension on withdrawal.

Before commencing treatment with lofexidine, baseline blood pressure should be measured and monitored over the first few days. If there is a significant drop in BP (systolic less than 90mmHg or 30mmHg below baseline), or pulse is below 55, lofexidine should be withheld. Treatment should be reviewed with the option to either continue at a reduced dose or discontinue.

Dose: Initially, 0.4–0.6mg twice daily, increased as necessary, to control withdrawal symptoms, in steps of 0.2–0.4mg daily, to a maximum total daily dose of 2.4mg . The total daily dose should be given in 2–4 divided doses, with one dose at bedtime to offset insomnia associated with opioid withdrawal. Treatment course should be 7–10 days, followed by a gradual withdrawal over 2–4 days.

Low, reducing doses of methadone (e.g. 15mg/10mg/5mg daily) may be given over the initial days of treatment with lofexidine as a cross-over period, to minimise withdrawal symptoms. This is only appropriate for patients currently taking methadone before detoxification.

Additional short-term medication may be required for nausea, stomach cramps, diarrhoea and insomnia.

Inpatient setting

✦ **Methadone**

Patients should have a starting dose assessment of methadone, over 48 hours as described above. The dose may then be reduced following a linear regime over 10 days.

✦ **Lofexidine**

(see community detoxification regimes above for more information)

Higher doses of lofexidine (up to the maximum daily dose of 2.4mg) may be given initially, particularly for patients with an average daily heroin use over 1/2g (or 30mg methadone equivalent). This is provided there is adequate monitoring of BP, pulse and adverse effects, and appropriate action can be taken in any such event. If there is a significant drop in BP or pulse, (systolic less than 90mmHg or 30mmHg below baseline, or pulse is below 55) lofexidine should be withheld until normal measurements are obtained and then re-introduced cautiously at a lower dose. In certain cases lofexidine may need to be discontinued and alternative detoxification treatment regimes considered.

The total daily dose should be given in four divided doses over the first two to three days with the full treatment course continuing for seven to ten days. This should then be followed by a gradual withdrawal over two to four days.

Additional short-term medication may be required for nausea, stomach cramps, diarrhoea and insomnia.

Opioid withdrawal scales

Objective scale – clinician assessed

Objectives	Absent / normal	Mild – moderate	Severe
Lactorrhoea	Absent	Eyes watery	Eyes streaming / wiping eyes
Rhinorrhoea	Absent	Sniffing	Profuse secretion (wiping nose)
Agitation	Absent	Fidgeting	Can't remain seated
Perspiration	Absent	Clammy skin	Beads of sweat
Piloerection	Absent	Barely palpable hairs standing up	Readily palpable, visible
Pulse rate (BPM)	< 80	≥ 80 but <100	≥ 100
Vomiting	Absent	Absent	Present
Shivering	Absent	Absent	Present
Yawning /10min	< 3	3–5	6 or more
Mydriasis	Normal ≤ 4mm	Dilated 4–6mm	Widely dilated >6mm

Subjective scale – patient reported

Subjectives	Absent	Mild	Moderate	Severe
Feeling sick				
Stomach cramps				
Muscle spasms/twitching				
Feelings of coldness				
Heart pounding				
Muscular tension				
Aches and pains				
Runny eyes				
Sweating				
Yawning				
Insomnia				

II) Alzheimer's disease and dementia

Drug treatment of Alzheimer's disease

Pathophysiology

✦ Destruction of cholinergic neurones, particularly in the cortex and hippocampus, is at least partly responsible for symptoms of Alzheimer's disease.

✦ Deficits in concentrations of choline acetyltransferase and acetylcholine have been observed and correlate with neuronal loss.

✦ Deficits in other neurotransmitters also occur.

✦ Neuronal death follows from the basic mechanisms of formation of plaques and tangles.

✦ Oxidative stress, cytotoxicity and inflammatory processes may be involved.

Mode of action

✦ Most drugs inhibit acetylcholinesterase and so prolong the activity of acetylcholine in the synapse.

✦ Some drugs are selective for acetylcholinesterase over butyrylcholinesterase. The latter is the soluble form of the enzyme found mainly in cardiac and smooth muscle. Inhibition of butyrylcholinesterase is not necessary for efficacy but may increase adverse effects.

✦ Some drugs may inhibit release of cytotoxic compounds from microglial cells.

✦ Other modes of action are possible.

Drug activity

Alzeimer's drugs may be shown to be effective in the following areas:

Global	Behavioural and neuropsychiatric
Cognitive	Effect on burden to caregiver
Functional	Disease modification

Drugs usually provide overall slowing of deterioration in global and cognitive domains and may also reduce functional loss and behavioural disturbance. There is considerable individual variation in response. No drug has been shown unequivocally to modify disease progression.

Summary of drug properties in Alzheimer's disease

| Drug | Mode of action | Efficacy in: | | | | | Tolerability |
		Global	Cognitive	Functional	Caregiver burden	Behavioural & neuro-psychiatric	
Tacrine	Acetylcholinesterase inhibitor	+	+	?	?	?	–
Donepezil	Acetylcholinesterase inhibitor	+	+	+	?	?	++ [1]
Rivastigmine	Acetylcholinesterase inhibitor	+	+	+	?	?	++ [1]
Galantamine	Acetylcholinesterase inhibitor	+	+	+	?	?	++ [1]

KEY: – poor
      + moderate
      ++ good

      ? evidence absent/equivocal

1. Tolerability dependent on dose and speed of titration.

Drug treatment of Alzheimer's disease – generic protocol

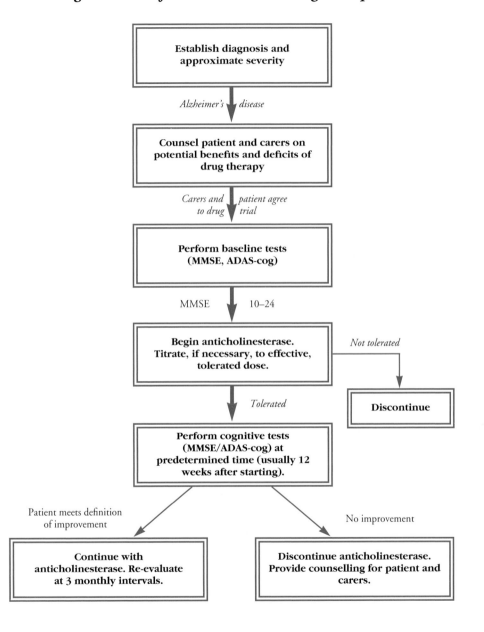

Establish diagnosis and approximate severity

Alzheimer's disease

Counsel patient and carers on potential benefits and deficits of drug therapy

Carers and patient agree to drug trial

Perform baseline tests (MMSE, ADAS-cog)

MMSE 10–24

Begin anticholinesterase. Titrate, if necessary, to effective, tolerated dose.

Not tolerated

Tolerated

Discontinue

Perform cognitive tests (MMSE/ADAS-cog) at predetermined time (usually 12 weeks after starting).

Patient meets definition of improvement

No improvement

Continue with anticholinesterase. Re-evaluate at 3 monthly intervals.

Discontinue anticholinesterase. Provide counselling for patient and carers.

Notes on protocol for drug treatment of Alzheimer's disease

✦ Diagnosis is best performed by a specialist, as are cognitive and functional tests.

✦ Counselling should include mention of the magnitude of effect likely, the possibility of adverse effects, and the likelihood of treatment failure.

✦ Commonly used cognitive tests include the Mini-Mental State Examination (MMSE) and the Alzheimer's Disease Assessment Scale – cognitive sub-scale (ADAS-cog). Many consider ADAS-cog unsuitable for routine clinical use. A number of other scales can be used.

✦ Anticholinesterase drugs have only been shown to be effective in patients with mild to moderate illness – usually a MMSE score of 10-24.

✦ Adverse effects include nausea, vomiting and diarrhoea. These effects are usually worse at higher doses and during rapid titration.

✦ "Improvement" is usually defined, somewhat arbitrarily, as a "worthwhile" change in MMSE and/or ADAS-cog. Exact values need to be defined locally, but are usually around 3 points on MMSE or −4 to −5 points on ADAS-cog at 3 months.

✦ An alternative definition of 'response' is simply a failure to deteriorate over 3–6 months. Most people with Alzheimer's show, if untreated, clear decline in cognition and functional ability over this period.

✦ Patients not meeting pre-determined criteria for improvement should be taken off drug therapy and provided with withdrawal counselling (include carers in this).

✦ Patients continuing after the first treatment evaluation are assumed to be "responders" and may continue with close monitoring. Note that deterioration is expected even in these responders and the decision to discontinue at some point must be taken on an individual basis.

✦ All drugs with anticholinergic effects should be avoided. Anticholinergic drugs may reduce the effect of anticholinesterases in all domains of efficacy: memory, activity, caregiver burden and behaviour may all be worsened.

Drugs to avoid:

Antipsychotics
–Chlorpromazine
–Clozapine
–Olanzapine
–Promazine
–Thioridazine

Anticholinergics
–Benzhexol
–Benztropine
–Hyoscine
–Orphenadrine
–Procyclidine

Antidepressants
–Tricyclic antidepressants
–Paroxetine
–MAOIs

References

Corey-Bloom J, Anand R, Veach J. (1998) A randomized trial evaluating the efficacy and safety of ENA 713 (rivastigmine tartrate), a new acetylcholinesterase inhibitor, in patients with mild to moderately severe Alzheimer's disease. *International Journal of Geriatric Psychopharmacology*, **1**, 55–65.

Cummings JL. (2000) Cholinesterase inhibitors: a new class of psychotropic compounds. *Am J Psychiatry*, **157**, 4–15.

Cummings JL, Askin-Edgar S. (2000) Evidence for psychotropic effects of acetylcholinesterase inhibitors. *CNS Drugs*, **13**, 385–395.

Hughes AM. Anticholinesterase in the treatment of Alzheimer's dementia – the first year's experience in Argyll & Clyde. Poster presented at 12th European College of Neuro-Psychopharmacology, September 1999, London, UK.

Jann MW. (1998) Pharmacology and clinical efficacy of cholinesterase inhibitors. *American Journal of Health-System Pharmacy* , **55 (suppl)**, S22–25.

Lovestone S, Graham N, Howard R. (1997) Guidelines on drug treatments for Alzheimer's disease. *Lancet*, **350**, 232–233.

Mantle D, Pickering AT, Perry EK. (2000) Medicinal plant extracts for the treatment of dementia: a review of their pharmacology, efficacy and tolerability. *CNS Drugs*, **13**, 201–213.

Matthews HP, Korbey J, Wilkinson DG, *et al.* First year results of donepezil use in a UK clinic for AD. Poster presented at the XI World congress of Psychiatry, August 1999, Hamburg, Germany.

Matthews HP, Korbey J, Wilkinson DG, *et al.* (1999) Donepezil in the treatment of Alzheimer's disease: results from the first eighteen months of a study in clinical practice in the UK. *Eur Neuropsychopharmacol* **9 (suppl 5)**, S327.

Rogers SL, Doody RS, Mohs RC, *et al.* (1998) Donepezil improves cognition and global function in Alzheimer's Disease. *Arch Intern Med*, **158**, 1021–1031.

Rogers SL, Farlow MR, Doody RS, *et al.* (1998) A 24-week, double-blind, placebo-controlled trial of donepezil in patients with Alzheimer's disease. *Neurology*, **50**, 136–145.

Rogers S, Friedhoff L. (1998) Long-term efficacy and safety of donepezil in the treatment of Alzheimer's disease: an interim analysis of the results of a US multicentre open label extension study. *Eur Neuropsychopharmacol*, **8**, 67–75

Winblad B, Engedal K, Soininen H, *et al.* Donepezil enhances global function, cognition and activities of daily living compared with placebo in a one-year double-blind trial in patients with mild to moderate Alzheimer's disease. Poster presented at the Ninth Congress of the International Psychogeriatric Association, August 1999, Vancouver, Canada.

III) Epilepsy

Treatment of psychiatric co-morbidity in people with epilepsy (PWE)

General recommendations for the use of antiepileptic drugs (AEDs)

✦   Choice of antiepileptic drugs (AEDs) should be made after considering the individual's epilepsy syndrome.

✦   Adverse psychotropic effects may be seen with all AEDs but, of the standard AEDs, are particularly common with phenobarbitone and primidone. Phenytoin may also have both positive and negative psychotropic effects and the clinician must be aware of its high protein binding, interactions, and non-linear kinetics in prescribing. Consider changing to carbamazepine or valproate, if clinically appropriate. Clobazam is generally better tolerated than 1,4 benzodiazepines and may be an effective adjunct, although tolerance develops in some 50% of patients. It is also effective as an anxiolytic, although this represents an off-licence use. Its use is restricted to treatment of epilepsy.

✦   The data with respect to the psychotropic effects of the newer AEDs are inconclusive, but lamotrigine and gabapentin may have some beneficial effects. Gabapentin has the advantage of very few drug interactions. Topiramate may cause adverse cognitive effects and must be titrated very slowly, over a period of months. Use of vigabatrin is severely limited because of neuropsychiatric toxicity and visual field defects and so BMJ guidelines should be followed if used. The extent of neuropsychiatric side effects and visual field defects with tiagabine need to be elucidated.

✦   It is useful to monitor total plasma concentrations of the older AEDs; the clinical role of plasma monitoring with the newer AEDs is yet to be established. Free AED levels in patients on phenytoin and sodium valproate are also useful, particularly if other protein-bound agents are being used concurrently.

✦   Consider the possible contribution of folate deficiency related to AED therapy to an individual's psychiatric presentation; RBC folate levels should be screened.

✦   Avoid polytherapy.

✦   Modified release preparations of carbamazepine and valproate are probably better tolerated and need to be taken less frequently.

✦   Pre-conception counselling is essential for women of child-bearing age.

Psychiatric co-morbidity in people with epilepsy (PWE)

General recommendations for the use of psychotropics

✦ It is important to start psychotropics at a low dose and then to increase slowly. Most seizures occur after a dose increase.

✦ Treat with the lowest effective dose and review regularly.

✦ All non-MAOI antidepressants may lower seizure threshold. SSRIs appear to do so less than TCAs but more data are needed. Fluoxetine has the advantage of being the best studied, but may increase AED levels - at times precipitously. Trazodone, citalopram and sertraline have the advantage of fewer drug interactions, although increases in AED levels may still occur and levels should be monitored. There are few data with respect to moclobemide, but it appears to be safe in epilepsy. Of the TCAs, there is some evidence that doxepin may be less epileptogenic than others and clomipramine more epileptogenic. Maprotiline, amoxapine and bupropion should be avoided. The use of MAOIs (except moclobemide) is not recommended when the patient is on carbamazepine therapy.

✦ ECT may increase seizure threshold. If clinically indicated, ECT is a reasonable altern-ative to consider in people with epilepsy. Other nonpharmacological treatments should also be considered.

✦ All antipsychotics may lower the seizure threshold. Of the newer antipsychotics, clozapine and zotepine should particularly be avoided. Haloperidol and fluphenazine may be less epileptogenic and chlorpromazine more epileptogenic than other standard antipsychotics. There are few data available on the effect of newer antipsychotics on seizure threshold, but risperidone and sulpiride appear to be well tolerated and have the advantage of fewer extrapyramidal adverse effects in patients who require long-term treatment.

✦ Consider drug interactions. Psychotropics may increase anticonvulsant plasma levels and anticonvulsants may lower psychotropic plasma levels. Monitor anticonvulsant plasma levels closely.

✦ Certain populations may be more susceptible to the epileptogenic potential of psy-chotropics and this should be taken into account when treating the elderly, people with mental disability or a history of head trauma, alcohol or drug abuse and those withdraw-ing from benzodiazepines or barbiturates.

Treatment of depression and psychosis in epilepsy

(Modified from McConnell and Duncan, 1998b)

Psychiatric presentation	Treatment
Peri-ictal depression	May be ictal or post-ictal affective symptoms; Inpatient admission for safety; Avoid antidepressants; Treat with optimisation of AEDs
Interictal depression	Moclobemide, SSRIs (fluoxetine, sertraline); Consider citalopram and trazodone; Consider ECT; Avoid maprotiline, amoxapine, mianserin, clomipramine; Consider role of AED adverse effects; Consider stigma, psychosocial issues, suicide risk; Avoid phenobarbitone, primidone, vigabatrin; Cognitive therapy and insight-oriented psychotherapy are useful
Bipolar disorder	Carbamazepine, sodium valproate Avoid phenobarbitone, primidone, vigabatrin; Consider ECT, lamotrigine, gabapentin Lithium is not contraindicated
Peri-ictal psychosis	Decide whether symptoms are ictal or post-ictal and treat accordingly; If ictal, avoid antipsychotics; Ictal psychosis needs to be treated urgently; Consider short-term haloperidol in post-ictal psychosis; Treat with optimisation of AEDs; Inpatient admission for safety
Interictal psychosis	Haloperidol, risperidone, sulpiride; Avoid clozapine, chlorpromazine and zotepine; Consider role of AED adverse effects; Avoid vigabatrin; Community support is important
Depression or psychosis related to AED therapy	Short-term psychotropics only as above; Withdraw offending agent and substitute with appropriate AED; Check folate and B12 levels

Treatment of anxiety disorders in epilepsy

(Modified from McConnell and Duncan, 1998b)

Psychiatric presentation	Treatment
Anxiety/ agoraphobia	Cognitive therapy; exposure; psychotherapy; education Psychotropics not generally indicated; Consider issues of self-esteem, driving, public perception, stigma Consider seizure and locus of control issues
Ictal panic/anxiety	Psychotropics not indicated; Best treated with optimisation of AED treatment; Consider clobazam
Generalised anxiety disorder	Propranolol; Avoid short-acting benzodiazepines; Consider clobazam, clonazepam, Avoid long-term benzodiazepines unless indicated for seizure control, Consider relaxation; biofeedback; cognitive therapy
Simple phobia	Psychotropics generally not indicated; exposure in vivo; Systematic desensitization; consider role of locus of control issues
Social phobia	Propranolol, MAOIs; avoid long-term benzodiazepines unless indicated for seizure control; anxiety management
Obsessive-compulsive disorder	Paroxetine, fluoxetine; avoid clomipramine; Consider clonazepam, if indicated, as well as for seizure control Consider thought stopping, exposure in vivo, response prevention
Panic disorder	Paroxetine, MAOIs, clonazepam, imipramine (low dose) Avoid long-term benzodiazepines unless indicated for seizure control; Cognitive therapy; relaxation exercises

Treatment of other psychiatric co-morbidity in epilepsy

(Modified from McConnell and Duncan, 1998b)

Psychiatric presentation	Treatment
Anorexia/bulimia	Fluoxetine; avoid clomipramine; Sodium valproate may be the preferred AED; Avoid topiramate (weight loss); Behavioural modification techniques; insight-oriented psychotherapy
Sexual dysfunction	Avoid tricyclics and SSRIs and venlafaxine; Consider switching to AED less likely to cause sexual dysfunction (e.g. lamotrigine); Consider role of AED adverse effects; Avoid carbamazepine, phenytoin, phenobarbitone, primidone; Treat underlying aetiology; Masters and Johnson techniques, education, involvement of partner and marital therapy are all useful
Cognitive dysfunction	Use AEDs with fewer cognitive effects (carbamazepine, lamotrigine); Treat underlying cause if possible; Treat concomitant depression, agitation; Consider role of AED adverse effects; Consider role of seizures, transient cognitive impairment (TCI); Avoid phenobarbitone, primidone, topiramate; Use of a diary as an aid to memory and involvement of family important; Milieu therapy can be helpful
Nonepileptic seizure-like events (NESLEs)	Treatment should be directed at underlying cause; Consider psychiatric, medical and neurological causes of NESLEs; Consider possibility of NESLEs coexisting with epileptic seizures; Biofeedback, cognitive behavioural therapy and psychotherapy are useful
Aggression	Carbamazepine; sodium valproate ? lithium; ? buspirone Consider role of AED adverse effects; avoid phenobarbitone, primidone; Behaviour modification and cognitive therapy are useful; Treat underlying cause of aggression
Attention deficit disorder	Treat with appropriate AED therapy in the first instance; Dexamphetamine and methylphenidate may be used if necessary; Consider role of AED adverse effects; Consider role of seizures, transient cognitive impairment (TCI); Avoid phenobarbitone, primidone; Behaviour modification techniques, supportive psychotherapy, family therapy and involvement of the school are all important

References

Aimard G, Vighetto A, Bret Ph, *et al.* (1989) Theraputique Neuropsychiatrique. Masson, Paris

Fogel BS, Schiffer RB. (eds) (1996) Neuropsychiatry. Williams & Wilkins, Baltimore, U.S.A.

Lishman A. (1998) Organic Psychiatry, Third Edition. Blackwell Science, Oxford, U.K.

McConnell HW, Snyder PJ. (1998) Psychiatric Co-morbidity in epilepsy: basic mechanisms, diagnosis and treatment. American Psychiatric Press, Washington DC, U.S.A.

Ruta DA. (1997) Neurology and guideline development. *Neurology*, **1**, 1–4.

Yudofsky SC, Hales RE. (eds) (1997) American Psychiatric Press Textbook of Neuropsychiatry. AP Press, Washington DC, USA

Use of standard antiepileptic drugs (AEDs)

(Modified from McConnell and Duncan, 1998a,b)

AED	Primary indications	Advantages	Disadvantages
Carbamazepine	Adjunctive or first line therapy in partial and generalised epilepsy (excluding absence and myoclonus); Lennox-Gastaut syndrome	Highly effective, inexpensive, well established; A drug of first choice in partial and generalised tonic-clonic seizures; Serum monitoring useful; Also useful as a mood stabiliser and for treatment of various pain conditions	Sedation, hyponatraemia, diplopia, ataxia, bone marrow dyscrasias, rash, Stevens-Johnson syndrome; Autoinduction; Be aware of possible cardiac toxicity in the elderly; Often poorly tolerated on initiation of therapy (transient); Many drug interactions
Clobazam	Adjunctive therapy in partial and generalised epilepsy; may be useful for intermittent therapy, one-off prophylaxis and catamenial seizures	Anxiolytic effects may be useful in concomitant panic disorder and other anxiety states; Excellent add-on therapy in treatment resistant patients	Sedation, agitation, disinhibition, withdrawal symptoms; Tolerance develops in up to half of patients, which severely limits its use
Clonazepam	Adjunctive therapy in partial and generalised epilepsy (including myoclonus and absence); Lennox-Gastaut syndrome; Infantile spasm; Status epilepticus	Some anxiolytic effects; Useful in children with refractory seizures; Some mood stabilising properties	Sedation particularly common, cognitive adverse effects, hyperactivity, aggression, withdrawal symptoms, ataxia, leucopenia; Usefulness limited by sedative and CNS effects and by tolerance
Ethosuximide	First-line or adjunctive therapy in generalised absence seizures. First line use declining.	A drug of first choice in absence seizures; Well established; Less hepatic toxicity than valproate in children; Serum monitoring useful	Gastric upset, ataxia, sedation, diplopia, psychosis, behavioural disturbance, rash, blood dyscrasias; Only effective in absence seizures

Drug			
Phenobarbitone (PB) and Primidone (PMD)	Previously used as adjunctive or first line therapy in partial and generalised epilepsy (excluding absence and myoclonus); status epilepticus (PB)	Inexpensive, effective, well established; IV preparation available for treatment of status epilepticus (PB); Serum monitoring useful but complicated by tolerance	Sedation, ataxia, hyperkinesis and learning difficulties (children), aggression, cognitive and sexual dysfunction, folate, vitamin K and D deficiency, withdrawal seizures; Not recommended in people with psychiatric co-morbidity
Phenytoin	Adjunctive or first line therapy in partial and generalised epilepsy (excluding absence and myoclonus); status epilepticus	Inexpensive, effective, well established; IV preparation available for treatment of status epilepticus; Serum monitoring mandatory	Sedation, gingival hyperplasia, hirsutism, blood dyscrasias, folate and Vitamin K deficiency, hypersensitivity, ataxia, dyskinesias, hepatitis; Many drug interactions; Non-linear kinetics
Sodium valproate	Adjunctive or first line therapy in partial and generalised epilepsy (including myoclonus and absence); Lennox-Gastaut syndrome; Juvenile myoclonic epilepsy	A drug of first choice in primary generalised epilepsies with the widest spectrum of efficacy of AEDs; Also effective as a mood stabiliser; Available as IV preparation	Weight gain, hair loss, severe hepatic toxicity in young children, blood dyscrasias, gastric upset, sedation, pancreatitis, tremor, hyperammonaemia; significant drug interaction with lamotrigine

Use of newer antiepileptic drugs (AEDs)

The newer AEDs are being increasingly used for first and second line therapy in many epilepsies. For example, lamotrigine has found an important role in the treatment of juvenile myoclonic epilepsy and many primary generalised syndromes in addition to its other indications. Gabapentin is well tolerated and has few interactions. Although it is used routinely in doses well above 3g overseas, its maximum dose recommendation in the BNF remains at 2400 mg daily. Gabapentin is also used off-licence overseas for various pain states particularly diabetic neuropathy and other neuropathic pain syndromes. Both gabapentin and lamotrigine are used off-licence as mood stabilisers. Topiramate initially developed problems with adverse effects related to its rapid titration which have been shown to improve somewhat with the slower schedule more recently introduced.

Concern over both the behavioural toxicity (particularly depression and psychosis) and the impairment in visual fields due to vigabatrin have caused many to reserve their use of this agent for very specific indications. It is still widely used in the UK for the treatment of infantile spasms and guidelines have recently been developed to assist the clinician in monitoring patients for the development of visual field defects and are available on the web for reference (www.bmj.com). The data are too few at this time to evaluate potential positive or negative behavioural side effects of tiagabine, launched in the UK in the later part of 1998. There have been reports of visual field loss occurring with tiagabine use which still need to be fully evaluated. The patients with these problems were also taking a variety of other medications.

Other AEDs, which should be mentioned here, include piracetam, which is useful for cerebral myoclonus and well tolerated. It is touted on the internet for its so-called 'smart drug' effects, but there is only anecdotal evidence as to its cognitive effects at present. Its sister drug levetiracetam appears effective for other types of seizures and is also well tolerated. Fos-phenytoin, a new parenteral preparation of phenytoin, has the advantage of being able to be administered intramuscularly and is safer and better tolerated than the previous preparations of parenteral phenytoin. Its role for the psychiatrist seeing patients with epilepsy remains to be elucidated but it appears very promising as an agent of choice for the treatment of status epilepticus in a psychiatric setting.

The guidelines presented here are meant to reflect the use of these agents in a psychiatric setting i.e. in the presence of psychiatric co-morbidity. The reader is referred to the guidelines of the Royal College of Physicians and the Institute of Neurology for treatment of adults with refractory epilepsy and to those of the Scottish Intercollegiate Guideline Network for treatment of seizures in a general neurology or medical setting. See also Crawford *et al.* (1999) for practice guidelines for women with epilepsy.

Use of newer antiepileptic drugs (AEDs)

Modified from McConnel and Duncan (1998a,b)

AED	Primary indications	Advantages	Disadvantages
Fosphenytoin	Status epilepticus	Parenteral formulation which can be given IM or IV; Better tolerated than older IV phenytoin parenteral preparations (less cardiac toxicity)	Probably has similar behavioural effect profile to phenytoin, but its exact role in a psychiatric setting remains to be elucidated
Gabapentin	Adjunctive therapy in refractory partial and secondarily generalised epilepsy; seizures occurring in porphyria	Few drug interactions; well tolerated; may be particularly useful in patients on multiple drugs or with hepatic impairment; may be titrated more quickly than other new AEDs; ? mood stabilising effects; effective in some pain states	Drowsiness, ataxia and nausea at high doses; seizure exacerbation reported; several case reports of behavioural disturbance in children with severe learning disabilities
Lamotrigine	Adjunctive or monotherapy in partial and generalised epilepsy; Lennox-Gastaut syndrome; Juvenile myoclonic epilepsy	Effective and well tolerated; few adverse behavioural or cognitive effects; wide spectrum of efficacy; may have some mood stabilising effects	Rash (may be severe). Serious rash more common in children; headache, ataxia, nausea, insomnia; Autoinduction; Drug interactions especially with standard AEDs
Piracetam	Cerebral myoclonus	Well tolerated; ? beneficial cognitive effects	Needs to be taken in large doses to be effective
Tiagabine	Add-on treatment of partial seizures with and without secondary generalisation	Few drug interactions; ? anxiolytic effects; ? usefulness in tardive dyskinesia	Dizziness, blurred vision, headache, rash, ? depression, ?psychosis; ? visual field effects
Topiramate	Adjunctive therapy in refractory partial and secondarily generalised epilepsy	Highly effective	Cognitive dysfunction, confusion, agitation, weight loss, dizziness, tremor, depression, renal calculi; Drug interactions with phenytoin and carbamazepine; Must be titrated slowly; Use limited by CNS toxicity
Vigabatrin	Adjunctive therapy in refractory partial and secondarily generalised epilepsy; Lennox-Gastaut syndrome; infantile spasms	Highly effective new AED for infantile spasms; Very few drug interactions	Sedation, dizziness, aggression, depression, psychosis, weight gain, ataxia, diarrhoea, case reports of irreversible peripheral field defects; Use severely limited by neuropsychiatric toxicity and by visual field deficits; Guidelines for monitoring of visual fields published by the BMJ (vol 317, p 1322) should be followed

Important interactions of antiepileptic drugs (AEDs) in psychiatry

(Modified from McConnell and Duncan, 1998b)

AED	Psychotropic interactions	Effects on other AEDs	Other interactions
Carbamazepine	CBZ may decrease levels of: antipsychotics (clozapine, haloperidol), TCAs, paroxetine, BZDs; CBZ levels may be increased by: viloxazine, TCAs, SSRIs; Presumed enhanced bone marrow toxicity with CBZ and clozapine; Increased risk of serotonin syndrome with SSRIs (case report); Theoretical increased risk of hypertensive crisis with MAOIs	Increased metabolism of PHT: will usually decrease, but may increase plasma levels of PHT; Decreased plasma levels of lamotrigine, tiagabine, topiramate and valproate; May decrease plasma levels of ethosuximide and primidone (by increased conversion to PHB)	Dextropropoxyphene, tramadol, erythromycin, isoniazid, warfarin, calcium channel blockers, lithium, danazol, corticosteroids, cyclosporin, diuretics, oral contraceptives, theophylline, thyroxine, paracetamol, cimetidine, vitamin D
Ethosuximide	None known	May increase plasma levels of PHT	Isoniazid, ? oral contraceptives
Gabapentin	None known	No known interactions with other AEDs; Isolated report of interaction with PHT	None known
Lamotrigine	None known	Case reports of increased plasma levels of 10-11, epoxide (CBZ metabolite), and of valproate	Paracetamol
Phenobarbitone	PHB may decrease levels of: antipsychotics, TCAs, paroxetine, BZDs; Additive sedative effects with antipsychotics, TCAs and BZDs; SSRIs may increase PHB levels; MAOIs may decrease PHB metabolism	Increased metabolism and decreased half-life of PHT, will usually decrease but may increase plasma levels of PHT; Decreased plasma levels of CBZ, clonazepam, lamotrigine, tiagabine and valproate; May decrease plasma levels of ethosuximide	Alcohol, disopyramide, warfarin, antibiotics, calcium channel blockers, thyroxine, corticosteroids, paracetamol, cyclosporin, theophylline, oral contraceptives, vitamin D

	Psychotropic drugs	AEDs	Other drugs
Phenytoin	PHT may decrease levels of: antipsychotics (clozapine), TCAs, paroxetine, BZDs; Phenothiazines may increase or decrease PHT levels; PHT levels may be increased by: TCAs, SSRIs; BZDs may increase or decrease PHT levels; Additive sedation with BZDs	Decreased half-life of PHB, increased or decreased plasma levels of PHB; Increased metabolism of BZDs, and increased clearance; Decreased plasma levels of lamotrigine, tiagabine, topiramate and valproate; Increased or decreased plasma levels of CBZ; Decreased plasma levels of ethosuximide and primidone (by increased conversion to PHB)	Aspirin, antacids, amiodarone, quinidine, disopyramide, mexiletine, antibiotics, warfarin, tolbutamide, antifungals, antimalarials, zidovudine, calcium channel blockers, corticosteroids, cyclosporin, methotrexate, disulfiram, carbonic anhydrase inhibitors, enteral foods, lithium, oral contraceptives, folate, theophylline, thyroxine, cimetidine, sucralfate, paracetamol, omeprazole, sulphinpyrazone, influenza vaccine, vitamin D
Tiagabine	Nefazodone and fluoxetine may increase tiagabine levels	May cause minor (10%) decreases in valproate levels	As tiagabine is metabolised by CYP3A4, erythromycin, grapefruit juice, and ketoconazole may increase tiagabine's plasma levels and rifampicin may reduce them
Topiramate	None known	May increase plasma levels of PHT	Oral contraceptives
Valproate	Case report of hepatotoxicity (chlorpromazine); SSRIs may increase valproate levels (case reports); Valproate may increase BZD levels; Increased and decreased clozapine levels reported	Increased PHB and lamotrigine levels; May decrease plasma levels of CBZ; May increase 10, 11 epoxide levels (CBZ metabolite); Increased or decreased plasma levels of PHT; May increase plasma levels of ethosuximide and primidone; May increase free tiagabine concentrations	Aspirin, cholestyramine, antimalarials, cimetidine
Vigabatrin	None known	Decreased plasma levels of PHT; May decrease plasma levels of PHB and primidone	None known

Abbreviations: SSRIs = selective serotonin reuptake inhibitors; TCAs = tricyclic antidepressants; MAOIs= monoamine oxidase inhibitors; BZD= benzodiazepines; PHB= phenobarbitone; CBZ= carbamazepine; PHT= phenytoin; AEDs= antiepileptic drugs
Note benzodiazepine interactions are listed under the psychotropic interaction column.

References

Appleton RE. (1998) Guideline may help in prescribing vigabatrin. *BMJ*, **317**, 1322.

Betts T. (1998) *Epilepsy, Psychiatry and Learning Difficulty*. Martin Dunitz, London, U.K.

Brown S, Betts T, Chadwick D, *et al*. (1993) An Epilepsy Needs Document. *Seizure*, **2**, 91–103.

Crawford P, Appleton R, Betts T. *et al*. (1999) Best Practice guidelines for the management of women with epilepsy. *Seizure*, **8**, 201–217.

Epilepsy Task Force. *Medical Treatment Guidelines*. Epilepsy Task Force/Joint Epilepsy Council, 1994

Fenwick PBC. (1988) Seizures, EEG discharges and Behaviour. In Epilepsy, Behaviour and Cognitive Function. MR Trimble and EH Reynolds (eds) John Wiley and Sons, Chichester, U.K., 51–66.

McConnell HW, Duncan D. (1998a) *Behavioural effects of antiepileptic drugs*. In: Psychiatric co-morbidity in epilepsy: basic mechanisms, diagnosis and treatment. McConnell H.W. and Snyder P.J. (eds.) American Psychiatric Press, Washington D.C., U.S.A., 205–244.

McConnell HW, Duncan D. (1998b) *The Treatment of Psychiatric Co-Morbidity in Epilepsy*. In: Psychiatric Co-morbidity in epilepsy: basic mechanisms, diagnosis and treatment. McConnell H.W. and Snyder P.J. (eds), Washington DC, American Psychiatric Press, U.S.A. Pg. 245–361.

McConnell H, Duncan D, Taylor D. (1997) Choice of neuroleptics in epilepsy. *Psych Bull*, **21**, 642–645.

McConnell H, Duncan D. The Use of Antiepileptic Drugs in psychiatry. In: R. Kerwin (ed): The Maudsley Textbook of Psychiatry (in press).

McConnell H, Duncan D. Psychiatric Co-morbidity in Epilepsy. In: R. Kerwin (ed): The Maudsley Textbook of Psychiatry (in press).

McConnell H, Snyder PJ. (1998) Electroencephalography in the elderly. In: P.Nussbaum (Ed.), Handbook of Neuropsychology and Aging. A volume in the *Critical Issues in Neuropsychology* series (E.E. Puente & C.R. Reynolds, Eds.). Plenum Press, New York, USA.

McConnell HW, Snyder PJ. (1998) Psychiatric Co-morbidity in epilepsy: basic mechanisms, diagnosis and treatment. American Psychiatric Press, Washington DC, U.S.A.

McConnell HW, Snyder PJ. The Clinicians's Perspective of Quality of Life in Epilepsy. In: Quality of Life in Epilepsy, G. Baker, A. Jacoby (eds), in press.

O'Connor R, Cox J, Couglan M. (1996) *Diagnosis and Management of Epilepsy in General Practice*. Irish College of General Practitioners, Dublin.

Report of Quality Standards Subcommittee of the American Academy of Neurology. (1998) Practice parameter: management issues for women with epilepsy (summary statement). *Neurology*, **51**, 944–947.

Scottish Intercollegiate Guideline Network (SIGN) (1997) *Diagnosis and Management of Adult Epilepsy in Primary and Secondary Care*, SIGN, Edinburgh

Shorvon S. (ed) (1996) The Treatment of Epilepsy. Blackwell Scientific, Oxford, U.K.

Snyder PJ, McConnell H. (1998) Epilepsy in the Elderly. In: P. Nussbaum (Ed.) Handbook of Neuropsychology and Aging. A volume in the Critical Issues in Neuropsychology series (A.E. Puente & C.R. Reynolds, Eds.). Plenum Press, New York, U.S.A.

Tomson T, Gram L, Sillanpaa M, *et al* (eds.) (1997) Epilepsy and Pregnancy. Rightson Medical Publishing, Petersfield, UK.

Trimble MR, Ring H, Schmitz B. (1996) Neuropsychiatric Aspects of Epilepsy. In: Fogel, B.S., Schiffer, R.B (eds) Neuropsychiatry. Williams & Wilkins, Baltimore. U.S.A.

Wallace H, Shorvon S, Hopkins A, *et al*. (1997) Adults with Poorly Controlled Epilepsy, Part I. Clinical Guidelines for Treatment, Royal College of Physicians of London.

Wilder BJ. (1998) Management of Epilepsy: Consensus Conference on Current Clinical Practice, *Neurology*, **51** (**5**) Suppl. 4.

IV) Gilles de la Tourette's Syndrome

✦ Gilles de la Tourette's syndrome (GTS) is characterised by the occurrence of motor and vocal tics and is usually of childhood onset. *Psychiatric co-morbidity* is common and may take a variety of forms. GTS is most frequently associated with obsessive-compulsive disorder (OCD), but may also be associated with other anxiety disorders, depression, and attention deficit disorder with hyperactivity (ADHD). Apart from a few case reports, there is no clear association of GTS with psychosis. The psychological and psychosocial reactions to this chronic neurological illness must also be considered in the treatment of GTS.

✦ The decision about whether to treat and, if so, what type of treatment to use, will depend on the degree to which the tics are interfering with the patient's ability to function productively.

✦ Start patients on the smallest dose of medication that is possible.

✦ Increase the dosage gradually paying close attention to the development of side effects as well as diminution of symptoms.

✦ Assure an adequate duration of any drug trial on sufficient dosage.

✦ Make changes in regimens slowly as sequences of single steps.

✦ When discontinuing medication be careful not to confuse withdrawal reactions with a need for more medication.

✦ Small doses of haloperidol (0.25-0.5 mg daily increasing by weekly intervals of 0.5 mg; usual maintenance dose: 2-3 mg) are useful in treating the *motor and vocal tics* associated with GTS. However, extrapyramidal symptoms, sedation and tardive dyskinesia are particular concerns with its use in this population. Sulpiride has fewer EPS, perhaps including tardive dyskinesia, and sedative effects and may be better tolerated by many. Gynaecomastia, galactorrhoea and menstrual problems have been reported with its use. Other antipsychotics may also be effective for treatment of tics, particularly fluphenazine and risperidone. Clonidine has the advantage of being well tolerated with no EPS and may be useful on its own or in augmenting the effects of antipsychotics. Small doses of pimozide are also effective in treating the tics in GTS, but its use requires ECG monitoring because of its cardiac effects. Dronabinol and other THC derivatives have been reported anecdotally to be of symptomatic assistance in GTS, but are not licensed in the UK for medical purposes.

✦ If *obsessive compulsive disorder* (OCD) is present, SSRIs are the treatment of choice. Currently only fluoxetine, paroxetine and fluvoxamine are licensed for use in OCD. Clomipramine is also effective but is less well tolerated. The use of buspirone for anxiety symptoms may increase motor tics. These same choices of antidepressants are useful in the treatment of *depression* in this population, as there are frequently obsessive-compulsive symptoms that are associated with the depressive illness. Other SSRIs or tricyclics may also be used safely. Behavioural therapy may be a useful adjunctive treatment.

✦ Clonidine is the treatment of choice if *ADHD* is present, as it may be effective in treating both the tics and the behavioural symptoms. Imipramine has been reported effective in this population as well and is preferable to the use of stimulants which may cause additional dykinesias. Methylphenidate and amphetamines are both effective in the treatment of ADHD, but regular monitoring for stimulant-induced dyskinesias is advised. Behavioural therapies are also very important in the treatment of ADHD in GTS.

Drugs of choice in Tourette's Syndrome

Condition	Treatment recommendations
Motor and vocal tics	Clonidine Haloperidol Pimozide* Sulpiride
Obsessive Compulsive Disorder	Clomipramine SSRIs (fluoxetine, paroxetine, fluvoxamine)
Attention Deficit Hyperactivity Disorder (ADHD)	Clonidine Dexamphetamine Imipramine Methylphenidate
Depression	Clomipramine SSRIs

* low dose only; ECG monitoring required

References

Chase TN, Friedhoff AJ, Cohen DJ. (1992) Tourette syndrome genetics, neurobiology and treatment. *Adv Neurol* **Vol.58** Raven Press, New York.

Comings DE. (1990) Tourette's Syndrome and Human Behavior. Hope Press, Duarte, CA, U.S.A.

Peterson BS. (1996) Considerations of natural history and pathophysiology in the psychopharmacology of Tourette's Syndrome. *J Clin Psychiatry*, **57**, 24–34.

Robertson, M. (1996) Gilles de la Tourette Syndrome and Obsessive-Compulsive Disorder. In: Fogel, B.S., Schiffer RB (eds) Neuropsychiatry. Williams & Wilkins, Baltimore. Pg. 827–870.

Sandor P. (1995) Clinical management of Tourette's syndrome and associated disorders. *Can J Psychiatry*, **40**, 577–583.

V) Head trauma and acquired brain injury (ABI)

General principles

◆ ABI can present with a variety of psychiatric symptoms.

◆ Complex partial seizures can produce a wide range of behavioural manifestations.

◆ Patients are often on other medical and CNS active drugs; beware of interactions.

◆ Avoid 'prn' medication (variable blood levels; may reinforce unwanted behaviours).

◆ Adverse effects from psychotropics are more common after ABI, particularly drug-induced akathisia, increased sensitivity to anticholinergic effects, decreased seizure threshold, increased propensity to sedation and confusion.

◆ Depression may be as common as 50% post ABI. The best predictor of depression is a previous history of depression. Always consider when deterioration is noted, particularly in early post-ABI recovery.

◆ Mania can be difficult to distinguish from early post ABI agitation until symptoms become more clearly defined. It may occur as a one-off episode in the absence of a previous history; an attempt to taper medication after the first episode should be considered.

◆ Dyscontrol and disinhibition are common and sometimes associated with orbital frontal and anterior temporal damage.

◆ Consider akathisia in the differential diagnosis of aggression, irritability or agitation in this population because of their susceptibility to this adverse effect.

◆ There are many factors contributing to the genesis of psychiatric comorbidity following head injury, including: premorbid personality, emotional impact of injury, circumstances of injury, repercussions of injury, iatrogenic factors, compensation issues, potential development of seizures, amount and location of injury (after Lishman, 1998).

◆ The degree and length of post-traumatic amnesia (PTA) relates to the development of psychiatric disability and intellectual impairment.

◆ If the PTA exceeds 24 hours, the likelihood of significant intellectual impairment increases markedly.

◆ Cognitive impairment, personality change, psychosis (schizophrenia, paranoid, affective), neurosis, and the ill-defined "post-traumatic syndrome" are all reported to occur following traumatic brain injury.

◆ Rehabilitation of intellectual impairment should involve the confidence and full co-operation of the patient, an optimistic approach, a graded programme, and careful attention to physical and psychological health. Retraining in attentional mechanisms may be beneficial and detection and treatment of underlying depression is important.

- One cannot underestimate the role of social adaptation and the effects on the family of head injury. Expressed Emotion ('EE') can be an important factor in the prediction of relapse and should be considered in the treatment plan of patients with head injury.

- EE has been hypothesised (McConnell and Duncan, 1998b) to relate to the social apraxia that may develop as a result of the patient losing the ability to recognise facial emotions in others and important social cues, usually due to right-sided injury or lesions of the amygdala. The subsequent interactions with the family may relate to the genesis of EE and should be considered in the family therapy sessions as part of rehabilitation.

- Choice of psychotropics should include consideration of epileptogenicity, potential interactions with other medications and the increased risk of adverse effects.

- Psychotropic medication should be started at a low dose and increased slowly, according to efficacy and tolerability.

References

Barrett K. (1991) Treating organic abulia with bromocriptine and lisuride. *J Neurol, Neurosurg Psychiatry*, **54**, 718–721.

Brooke MM, Patterson DR, Questad KA, *et al.* (1992) The treatment of agitation during initial hospitalisation after traumatic brain injury. *Arch Phys Med Rehab*, **73**, 917–921.

Feeney DM, Gonzalez A, Law WA. (1982) Amphetamine, haloperidol and experience interact to affect rate of recovery after motor cortex injury. *Science*, **217**, 855–857.

Geracioti TD. (1994) Valproic acid treatment of episodic explosiveness related to brain injury. *J Clin Psychiatry*, **55**, 416–417.

Greendyke RM, Kanter DR. (1986) Therapeutic effects of pindolol on behavioural disturbances associated with organic brain disease: A double-blind study. *J Clin Psychiatry*, **47**, 423–426.

Lewin J, Sumners D. (1992) Successful treatment of episodic dyscontrol with carbamazepine. *Br J Psychiatry*, **161**, 261–262.

Lishman WA. (1998) Organic Psychiatry, Third Edition. Blackwell Science: London, UK.

McConnell HW, Duncan D. (1998) *The Treatment of Psychiatric Co-Morbidity in Epilepsy*. In: Psychiatric Co-morbidity in epilepsy: basic mechanisms, diagnosis and treatment. McConnell H.W. and Snyder P.J. (eds), Washington DC, American Psychiatric Press, U.S.A. Pg. 245–361.

Pourcher E, Filteau MJ, Bouchard RH, *et al.* (1994) Efficacy of the combination of buspirone and carbamazepine in early posttraumatic delirium. *Am J Psychiatry*, **151**, 150–151.

Robinson RG, Jorge R. (1994) Mood Disorders, in *Neuropsychiatry of Traumatic Brain Injury*, (Eds) J.M. Silver, S.C. Yudofsky and R.E. Hale. American Psychiatry Press Inc: Washington, U.S.A.

Treatment of psychiatric comorbidity following acquired brain injury

Condition	Recommended treatment
Abulia	❖ Exclude other aetiologies e.g. depression, sedation from antipsychotics, negative symptoms of schizophrenia-like psychosis ❖ Behavioural interventions ❖ Dopamine agonists such as bromocriptine or lisuride may occasionally be helpful in the hands of a clinician experienced with their use
Bipolar disorder	❖ Valproate or antipsychotics (haloperidol) may be useful in acute stages ❖ Carbamazepine and lithium, initiated gradually, may be used for prophylaxis, if indicated; however, episodes of mania/agitation can occur as isolated events and do not necessarily recur
Delirium	❖ General supportive care (consider metabolic causes, drugs or withdrawal syndromes as a cause of confusion) ❖ Short term sedation with clonazepam/chlormethiazole ❖ Consider risperidone or sulpiride if an antipsychotic is needed ❖ Carbamazepine and buspirone may also be considered
Depression	❖ Social support and multidisciplinary approach is very important; involving relatives where possible ❖ Cognitive and behavioural treatment should be used as adjunctive therapy ❖ SSRIs treatment of choice ❖ ECT to be avoided in first 6 months post injury
Dyscontrol / disinhibition	❖ Exclude other psychiatric pathology/epilepsy ❖ Mainly behavioural assessments to identify triggers etc ❖ Drugs may be useful e.g. carbamazepine and beta blockers (Lewin & Sumners,1992; Greendyke et al, 1986) ❖ Benzodiazepines may worsen symptoms
Psychosis	❖ Most post ABI psychoses respond well to antipsychotic agents, but patients are more likely to suffer adverse effects ❖ Sulpiride may be drug of choice; best to use less epileptogenic antipsychotics (see section above) ❖ Assess response in the usual way after 6-8 week trial ❖ Carbamazepine has been reported to be effective in some cases
Social apraxia	❖ Social apraxia has been hypothesised (McConnell and Duncan, 1998b) to be related to an inability to pick up social cues and to recognise facial emotions due usually to right-sided lesions and/or to damage to the amygdala ❖ Social apraxia often confused with personality issues, but important to recognise as represents a treatable cause of such behavioural and social problems ❖ Such a loss of ability to recognise facial features and key social cues is best approached from a practical, skill-based perspective using communication skills training, group therapy and anger management.

VI) Multiple Sclerosis

✦ *Depression* is a common occurrence in patients with multiple sclerosis (MS), occurring with a point prevalence of approximately 27%. Depression may be due to a psychological reaction to a chronic neurological illness, related to the illness itself or to treatment with beta interferon, ACTH or steroids. Pathological laughter and pathological crying may also occur and be independent of the underlying emotional state of the individual. *Apathy states* and *abulia* as well as disorders of *lability of affect* may occur. Personality changes, intellectual impairment and euphoria are also common in patients with MS. There are also some case reports of *psychosis* in MS. There are few data available to suggest *treatment strategies* in psychiatric co-morbidity in MS. Below are some general considerations for prescribing of psychotropics in this population.

✦ Tricyclics are effective in treating depression in this disorder, but are not well tolerated, with very high drop out rates related to anticholinergic effects. SSRIs are effective, at least in one retrospective study with sertraline, and appear to be well tolerated. Sertraline (and probably other SSRIs) are thus preferred as antidepressants of choice.

✦ If psychiatric effects are felt related to medical therapy of MS, treatment should be directed at removal or reduction in dosage of the causal agent. Beta–interferon has been associated with adverse psychiatric effects, particularly depression and lethargy. Side effects are generally dose related. Steroids and baclofen (for spasticity) have also been associated with depression and psychosis and neither are well tolerated in abrupt withdrawal.

✦ There are recent reports of cannabinoids being effective for 'well-being' and for analgesia in MS. There is currently, however, no licence for the medical use of this class of drugs in the UK.

✦ There are few data available as to choice of antipsychotics in MS. Drugs that have fewer EPS and anticholinergic effects (e.g. olanzapine, risperidone) may, however, be better tolerated in this population.

References

Mahler ME. (1992) Behavioral manifestations associated with Multiple Sclerosis. *Psychiat Clin North Am,* **15**, 427–437.

Scott TF, Allen D, Price TRP, *et al.* (1996) Characterization of major depression symptoms in Multiple Sclerosis patients. *J Neuropsychiatry Clin Neurosci* **8**, 318–323.

Scott T, Nussbaum P, McConnell H, *et al.* (1996) Measurement of Treatment Response to Sertraline in Depressed Multiple Sclerosis Patients Using The Carroll Scale. *Neurology Research,* **7**, 421–422.

VII) Parkinson's Disease

◆ *Depression* is a common manifestation of Parkinson's disease (PD) occurring in about 1/3 of patients in the community and about 1/2 of hospital patients. The characteristic loss of facial expression, psychomotor retardation, alterations in gait and changes in speech, typical of early PD, should not be mistaken for a sign of depression, however, and a careful mental state examination should clarify the issue. Depression and anhedonia must be present to confirm the diagnosis of depression. Note that an amotivational syndrome occurs in one third of patients and this should be differentiated from depression. *Mania*, on the other hand, is rare in PD and is usually due to dopaminergic treatment when present.

◆ *Tricyclics* are effective in treating depression in PD and may also be helpful from the stand-point of EPS by virtue of their anticholinergic activity; however, tricyclics may also uncommonly cause EPS and may impair absorption of levodopa. The anticholinergic activity may also increase confusion in the elderly. Of the tricyclics, lofepramine has the advantage of fewer adverse cardiac effects and less serotonergic activity. Nortriptyline has been shown to be effective and well tolerated in one double-blind placebo-controlled study. Imipramine and desipramine (now discontinued) have also been found to be efficacious in treating depression in PD. Amoxapine should be avoided because of its potential to cause Pakinsonism.

◆ *SSRIs* may be effective in treating depression associated with PD, although there have been no controlled trials and there have been case reports of fluoxetine and paroxetine exacerbating the motor symptoms in PD. All SSRIs have tremor as a common adverse effect. SSRIs and clomipramine should not be used with selegiline as there are reports of serotonergic reactions as well as of increased EPS with this combination.

◆ *MAOIs* (including *moclobemide*) interact with levodopa, causing hypertensive crisis and should thus be avoided in PD. They also may interact with selegiline and this combination is also not recommended. If selegiline is used with moclobemide, full MAO inhibition may occur and full MAOI dietary precautions are necessary. Selegiline itself may have some anti-depressant effects as well as effects on the movement disorder in PD.

◆ Of the *mood stabilising agents*, sodium valproate and lithium can both cause tremor independently of PD and this may be difficult to differentiate from the primary tremor associated with PD. Sodium valproate has also been associated with other EPS. Consider the possibility of these agents affecting the tremor in PD if it is exacerbated after starting them or increasing their dosage, even if serum levels are in the 'therapeutic' range. Carbamazepine is preferred as a mood stabiliser in PD.

◆ *Electroconvulsive therapy* (ECT) is a useful treatment for depression in PD and may also alleviate the parkinsonian symptoms, albeit temporarily.

◆ *Psychosis* occurs in 20-30% of patients. It is frequently caused by treatment of PD and its therapy should, in the first instance be directed at reducing or stopping the most recently added antiparkinsonian agent. Otherwise antiparkinsonian agents should be reduced or discontinued in the following order: anticholinergics, MAO-B inhibitors, amantadine, dopamine receptor agonists. If there is no improvement in psychotic symptoms, then levodopa should be gradually reduced. Administering levodopa after food intake may slow its absorption and diminish its adverse psychiatric effects. If there is still no improvement in symptoms, olanzapine or clozapine should be added with reassessment of motor status. If an aggravation of motor symptoms occurs, antiparkinsonian agents should be cautiously reintroduced in the reverse order given above.

✦ Avoid use of *antipsychotics* with a particularly high propensity to cause extrapyramidal side effects (EPS) e.g. haloperidol, phenothiazines. Consider the use of atypical antipsychotics which may have fewer EPS e.g. clozapine, olanzapine, quetiapine. Of these, clozapine has been most studied and may have some beneficial effects on the EPS of PD in addition to effectively treating the psychosis. It should be noted, however, that the elderly may be more predisposed to agranulocytosis with clozapine. Clozapine is also licensed only for the treatment of refractory schizophrenia and, as its prescribing is tightly controlled, it may be difficult to get approval for its use in a non-schizophrenic population. There are conflicting reports of the use of risperidone, with some reporting this to be effective and others reporting exacerbation of EPS with its use in PD. Olanzapine has been found effective and well tolerated and quetiapine has been used with good results.

✦ *Dopamine dyskinesias* (DD) are very common in patients treated with long-term levodopa and may also occur after only 4 weeks of therapy. This must be differentiated from tardive dyskinesia in the case of patients treated with concomitant antipsychotics.

✦ *Dementia* occurs up to 10 times more frequently in patients with PD, depending on the particular parkinsonian syndrome. Aggressive treatment of depression and minimising the use of anticholinergics may help to reduce cognitive deficits. Conversely, cholinomimetic agents may be of benefit.

✦ *Anxiety* is also a common occurrence in PD. It occurs early in the course of PD and may be associated with a depressive illness. If benzodiazepines are used, it should be noted that they may occasionally antagonise the effects of levodopa.

Psychotropic group	Recommendations
Antidepressants	Lofepramine Nortriptyline
Antipsychotics	Clozapine Olanzapine ? Quetiapine
Mood stabilisers	Carbamazepine

References

Cole SA, Woodard JL, Juncos JL, *et al.* (1996) Depression and disability in Parkinson's Disease. *J Neuropsychiatry Clin Neurosci,* **8**, 20–25.

Factor SA, Molho ES, Brown DL. (1995) Combined clozapine and electroconvulsive therapy for the treatment of drug-induced psychosis in Parkinson's disease. *J Neuropsychiatry Clin Neurosci,* **7**, 304–307.

Hegeman-Richard I, Schiffer RB, Kurlan R. (1996) Anxiety and Parkinson's Disease. *J Neuropsychiatry Clin Neurosci,* **8**, 383–392.

Juncos J, Yeung P, Sweitzer D. Quetiapine improves Psychotic Symptoms Associated with Parkinson disease. Poster presented at APA Annual Meeting, May 1999, Washington DC.

Klaassen T, Verhey FRJ, Sneijders GHJM, *et al.* (1995) Treatment of depression in Parkinson's Disease: a meta-analysis. *J Neuropsychiatry Clin Neurosci* **7**, 281–286.

Mendis T, Barclay CL, Mohr E. (1996) Drug-induced psychosis in Parkinson's Disease: a review of management. *CNS Drugs,* **5**, 166–174.

Musser WS, Akil M. (1996) Clozapine as a treatment for psychosis in Parkinson' Disease: A review. *J Neuropsychiatry Clin Neurosci,* **8**, 1–9.

Parsa MA and Bastani B. (1998) Quetiapine (Seroquel) in the treatment of psychosis in patients with Parkinson's disease. *J Neuropsychiatry Clin Neurosci,* **10**, 216–219.

Pfeiffer C, Wagner ML. (1994) Clozapine therapy for Parkinson's disease and other movement disorders. *Am J Hosp Pharm,* **51**, 3047–3053.

Wagner ML, Defilippi JL, Menza MA, *et al.* (1996) Clozapine for the treatment of psychosis in Parkinson's Disease: chart review of 49 patients. *Journal of Neuropsychiatry,* **8**, 276–280.

Wolters ECh, Jansen ENH, Tuynman-Qua HG, *et al.* (1996) Olanzapine in the treatment of dopaminomimetic psychosis in patients with Parkinson's Disease. *Neurology,* **47**, 1085–1087.

VIII) Porphyria

✦ The porphyrias are associated with a variety of neuropsychiatric manifestations, including seizures, psychosis and affective symptoms. They may be associated with abdominal pain and/or with a discolouration of urine during attacks, but these features may also be absent.

✦ There are many types of porphyrias and the diagnostic tests for evaluation and drugs which exacerbate each syndrome are different. Note also the difficulties inherent in diagnosing acute porphyria; obtaining bloods and urines during the acute symptomatic phase may be important.

✦ Acute porphyria may be exacerbated by many drugs and an acute exacerbation is treated with haemarginate. Vomiting can be treated with promazine and pain can be treated with pethidine, dihydrocodeine or morphine.

✦ Gabapentin and sodium valproate are the safer AEDs.

✦ Close attention to electrolytes may be important, particularly if vomiting is present. The following psychotropics are to be avoided in porphyria as they have been associated with precipitating acute attacks:

–amphetamines
– tricyclic and related antidepressants (except amitriptyline and lofepramine)
– monoamine oxidase inhibitors (MAOIs)   *– carbamazepine*
– benzodiazepines (?)   *– lamotrigine*
– barbiturates   *–phenytoin*

Advice on the safety of medical and psychiatric therapies in this disorder is available from the National Porphyria Service in the UK (029 20 742 979). The clinician is advised to telephone with concerns about both diagnosis and treatment before starting treatment in known or suspected porphyria as information about possible adverse effects is constantly changing. This Centre has produced a bulletin on this topic and have available a list of drugs which are considered safe in the acute porphyrias.

Psychotropic group	Recommendations
Antidepressants	Amitriptyline Fluoxetine Lofepramine
Antipsychotics	Chlorpromazine Droperidol Haloperidol Trifluoperazine
Mood stabilisers	Lithium Sodium valproate

References

Crimlisk HL. (1997). The little imitator B porphyria: a neuropsychiatric disorder. *J Neurol Neurosurg Psychiatry*, **62**, 319–328.

Lishman WA. (1998) Organic Psychiatry Third Edition, Blackwell Science, Oxford, pp. 567–569.

IX) Stroke

✦ Depression is a common occurrence following a stroke, affecting approximately one third of patients. The greatest risk is within the first two years of a stroke and those with left – anterior or right – posterior lesions are at greater risk. Those with non-fluent aphasia are also at greater risk, although it is not clear whether this is a causal relationship or whether it is an independent outcome arising from damage in the same region. Left hemisphere lesions may also be related to the development of cognitive impairment with depression. Depression may relate to a psychological reaction to the illness and/or to the site of brain injury itself or nature and degree of disability. Other risk factors for the development of depression include a personal or family history of depression, and the presence of subcortical atrophy preceding the stroke.

✦ The choice of antidepressant following a stroke is dependent on the age of the patient, the potential for epileptogenicity of the lesion, the use of anticoagulant therapy or of other cardiac drugs, and the efficacy of the antidepressant in this population. Because many patients with cerebrovascular disease are also elderly and have concomitant cardiac disease, the recommendations set out in both these sections generally apply to this population as well. Consideration of the epileptogenic potential of psychotropics is also important, as the brain injury sustained as a result of the stroke puts the patient at an increased risk for development of seizures and an antidepressant with low epileptogenic potential is also preferred (see section on Epilepsy). As concerns efficacy, there are few data available, but studies have been done showing nortriptyline, citalopram and trazodone to be effective in treating post-stroke depression. Tricyclics, however, are often poorly tolerated in this population and their anticholinergic effects, adverse cardiac profile and epileptogenicity make them a less desirable choice for the treatment of post-stroke depression. SSRIs and moclobemide are thus the antidepressants of choice in this population.

✦ Drug interactions are an important consideration in the selection of psychotropics in this population. Many patients will be on aspirin which will increase the free plasma concentrations of highly protein-bound drugs (e.g. sodium valproate, fluoxetine, paroxetine, sertraline amongst others). Patients on anticoagulant therapy with warfarin (e.g. those at risk of embolic stroke, atrial fibrillation) present a particular problem in the choice of antidepressants because of potential interactions which may increase the INR and cause potentially serious haemhorragic complications. These are summarised in the following table.

✦ Citalopram may be less likely than nefazodone and sertraline to interact with warfarin. Fluoxetine and fluvoxamine appear to have the highest potential of the antidepressants for interactions. Interactions of other cardiac medications should also be considered.

Psychotropic interactions with warfarin

(Modified from Duncan et al, 1998 and Greenblatt et al, 1998)

Antidepressant	Mechanisms of potential interaction
SSRIs	Fluoxetine: Highly protein bound; moderate inhibitor of CYP2C9, CYP2C19 and CYP3A;? substrate at CYP2C9 Fluvoxamine: Not highly protein bound; potent inhibitor of CYP1A2 and CYP2C19; moderate inhibitor of CYP2C9 and CYP3A; ? substrate at CYP1A2 Paroxetine: Highly protein bound Sertraline: Highly protein bound; ? substrate at CYP2C9 and CYP3A; minor to moderate inhibitor of CYP2C19 Citalopram: Not highly protein bound; not a major inhibitor of isozymes; substrate at CYP2C19 and CYP3A
Nefazodone	Highly protein bound; potent inhibitor of CYP3A; substrate at CYP3A
Trazodone	Highly protein bound; Substrate at CYP1A2; P450 metabolism poorly understood; single case report
Venlafaxine	Not highly protein bound; substrate at CYP2C19 and CYP3A; no interaction studies available
Moclobemide	Not highly protein bound;? inhibitor of CYP1A2 and CYP2C19; substrate at CYP2C19; no interaction studies available
MAOIs (tranylcypromine)	May inhibit cytochrome P450 (inhibits CYP2C19); extent of protein binding is not known
TCAs	Highly protein bound; substrate at CYP1A2, CYP2C19, and/or CYP3A; anticholinergic effects may slow gastric motility and thus increase time available for dissolution and absorption of warfarin

✦ Pathological crying ('emotional incontinence', 'pseudobulbar affect') may occur after stroke and is, characteristically, unrelated to the inner emotional state of the individual. Nortriptyline, amitriptyline and citalopram have been shown to alleviate pathological crying after stroke.

✦ Post-stroke apathy may occur independently of depression following stroke and may be difficult to differentiate from an affective illness.

✦ Mania is a rare (<1%) manifestation of acute stroke and may occur more frequently in right orbitofrontal or basotemporal lesions or through diaschisis. There are no controlled trials of the treatment of bipolar disorder or of mania following stroke. Because of the epileptogenic potential of the lesion following stroke, however, sodium valproate and carbamazepine may be preferable to lithium in treating this population. If carbamazepine is used in patients with concomitant cardiac disease, a baseline ECG should be obtained as well as regular cardiac monitoring.

- *Post-stroke psychosis* is also relatively uncommon and may occur as part of a delirium or as an hallucinosis. The same considerations for the choice of antipsychotics apply as in the elderly and in patients with epilepsy and cardiac disease. Other psychiatric manifestations following stroke include generalised *anxiety* (often associated with depression), *anosognosia* (especially in right hemisphere lesions), and the so-called '*catastrophic reaction*' seen with anterior cortical lesions and, at times, with aphasia. A catastrophic reaction occurs in about 20% of stroke patients and may be indicative of a behavioural or emotional expression of an underlying depression associated with anterior cortical or subcortical damage.

SSRIs, the half-lives of sertraline and citalopram are prolonged in the elderly. If a tricyclic antidepressant is required, nortriptyline may be better tolerated. Amoxapine should be avoided because of its potential for causing EPS in this at risk population, as should tricyclics with a greater degree of anticholinergic activity. Trazodone and nefazodone may also be antidepressants of choice because they have fewer cardiac and anticholinergic effects. Orthostatic hypotension may need to be monitored, however. MAOIs should be avoided because of their propensity to cause orthostatic hypotension and because the dietary restrictions may be difficult to follow for some.

- *Electroconvulsive therapy (ECT)* is a safe and effective treatment option in this population for severe depression and for mania and may be better tolerated than pharmacotherapy in some patients.

- For late-onset *bipolar disorder*, lithium appears to be as effective as in early-onset cases, but long-term follow-up studies have not been done to date. Lithium toxicity may occur at levels that would be considered 'therapeutic' in younger patients. Lithium clearance is reduced in the elderly and doses may be upto 50% lower. Of AED mood stabilisers, carbamazepine has more adverse cardiac effects and needs to be monitored with ECGs in the elderly and sodium valproate may thus be preferred. The half-life of valproate may be longer in the elderly and the free fraction may also be increased.

- The elderly are much more susceptible to the extrapyramidal symptoms (EPS) of *antipsychotics* as well as to the orthostatic hypotension and anticholinergic effects of these agents. When indicated they should be used in much lower doses (generally one half to one third of doses in younger adults) and titrated more slowly with frequent monitoring. It is useful to monitor the elderly for Parkinsonian side effects and for tardive dyskinesia on a three monthly basis and more frequently at the onset of therapy or when making dose adjustments. Clozapine may be associated with an increased incidence of agranulocytosis in the elderly and anecdotally has not been thought as effective as in younger adults. Sertindole should not be used in the elderly because of its cardiac effects and drug interactions. Risperidone may be used in the elderly, but its half life may be increased and blood pressure should be monitored. The lesser cardiac, anticholinergic and extrapyramidal effects of sulpiride and olanzapine make these drugs of choice in this population.

- *Benzodiazepines* and *drugs with a high degree of anticholinergic activity* should be avoided.

Use of psychotropics following stroke

Psychotropic classification	Recommended drugs
Antidepressants	Moclobemide SSRIs
Antipsychotics	Olanzapine Risperidone Sulpiride
Mood stabilisers	Lithium Sodium Valproate

References

Absher JR, Toole JF. (1996) Neurobehavioral features of cerebrovascular disease. In: Fogel BS, Schiffer RB (eds) *Neuropsychiatry*. Williams & Wilkins, Baltimore, Pg 895–912.

Duncan D, Sayal K, McConnell H, *et al* (1998) Antidepressant interactions with warfarin. *Int Clin Psychopharmacol*, **13**, 87–94.

Graff-Radford NR, Biller J. (1992) Behavioral neurology and stroke. *Psychiatr Clin North Am*, **15**, 415–425.

Greenblatt DJ, von Moltke LL, Harmatz JS, *et al*. (1998) Drug interactions with newer antidepressants: role of human cytochromes P450. *J Clin Psychiatry*, **59 (suppl 15)**, 19–27.

House A. (1996) Depression associated with stroke. *J Neuropsychiatry Clin Neurosci*, **8**, 454-457.

VI

Management of
Medical/Psychiatric
Emergencies

Management of simple paracetamol poisoning

This protocol is suitable for poisoning with paracetamol alone. Do not use this protocol if you suspect another substance has been taken in excess

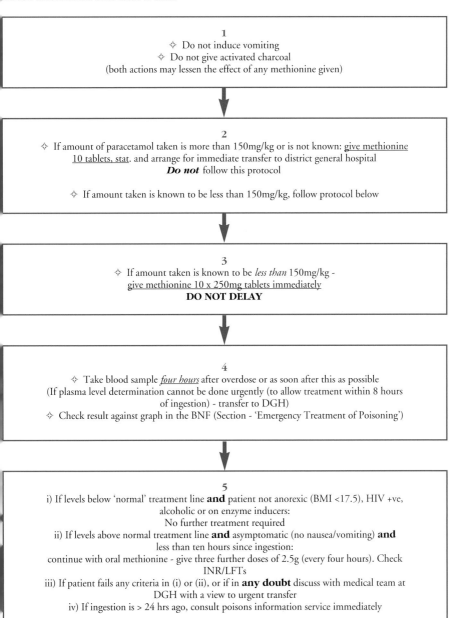

1
- ✧ Do not induce vomiting
- ✧ Do not give activated charcoal
(both actions may lessen the effect of any methionine given)

2
- ✧ If amount of paracetamol taken is more than 150mg/kg or is not known: <u>give methionine 10 tablets, stat.</u> and arrange for immediate transfer to district general hospital
Do not follow this protocol

- ✧ If amount taken is known to be less than 150mg/kg, follow protocol below

3
- ✧ If amount taken is known to be *less than* 150mg/kg -
<u>give methionine 10 x 250mg tablets immediately</u>
DO NOT DELAY

4
- ✧ Take blood sample <u>*four hours*</u> after overdose or as soon after this as possible
(If plasma level determination cannot be done urgently (to allow treatment within 8 hours of ingestion) - transfer to DGH)
- ✧ Check result against graph in the BNF (Section - 'Emergency Treatment of Poisoning')

5
i) If levels below 'normal' treatment line **and** patient not anorexic (BMI <17.5), HIV +ve, alcoholic or on enzyme inducers:
No further treatment required
ii) If levels above normal treatment line **and** asymptomatic (no nausea/vomiting) **and** less than ten hours since ingestion:
continue with oral methionine - give three further doses of 2.5g (every four hours). Check INR/LFTs
iii) If patient fails any criteria in (i) or (ii), or if in **any doubt** discuss with medical team at DGH with a view to urgent transfer
iv) If ingestion is > 24 hrs ago, consult poisons information service immediately

Acute disturbed or violent behaviour

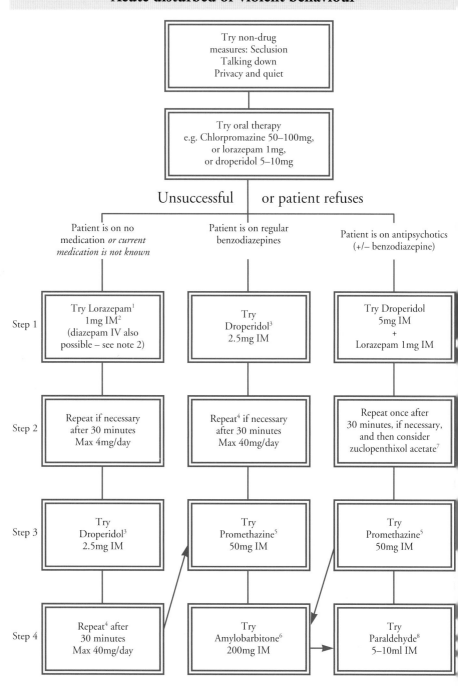

Try non-drug
measures: Seclusion
Talking down
Privacy and quiet

Try oral therapy
e.g. Chlorpromazine 50–100mg,
or lorazepam 1mg,
or droperidol 5–10mg

Unsuccessful | or patient refuses

Patient is on no medication *or current medication is not known*

Patient is on regular benzodiazepines

Patient is on antipsychotics (+/– benzodiazepine)

Step 1
Try Lorazepam[1] 1mg IM[2] (diazepam IV also possible – see note 2)

Try Droperidol[3] 2.5mg IM

Try Droperidol 5mg IM + Lorazepam 1mg IM

Step 2
Repeat if necessary after 30 minutes Max 4mg/day

Repeat[4] if necessary after 30 minutes Max 40mg/day

Repeat once after 30 minutes, if necessary, and then consider zuclopenthixol acetate[7]

Step 3
Try Droperidol[3] 2.5mg IM

Try Promethazine[5] 50mg IM

Try Promethazine[5] 50mg IM

Step 4
Repeat[4] after 30 minutes Max 40mg/day

Try Amylobarbitone[6] 200mg IM

Try Paraldehyde[8] 5–10ml IM

Notes

1. Mix lorazepam 1:1 with water for injections before injecting. If lorazepam is not available, consider using midazolam IM.
2. Have flumazenil available to reverse the effects of lorazepam. (Monitor respiratory rate – give flumazenil if rate falls below 10/min.) Consider intravenous route if 3 doses of lorazepam fail to have any effect.

   Some centres use IV benzodiazepines (diazepam (5–10mg) as Diazemuls is often used). IV therapy may be used instead of IM when a very rapid effect is required. IV therapy also ensures near immediate delivery of the drug to its site of action and effectively avoids the danger of inadvertent accumulation of slowly absorbed IM doses. Note also that IV doses can be repeated after only 5–10 minutes if no effect is observed.

3. Caution in patients who have never before received neuroleptics. Have procyclidine IM available. Consider giving 5mg at the same time as droperidol.
4. If 2.5mg IM droperidol is ineffective after 30 minutes, try 5mg and then 10mg, if necessary. Consider giving intravenously (5mg–10mg) if three IM doses have no effect.
5. Promethazine has a slow onset of action but is often an effective sedative. Dilution is not required before IM injection. May be repeated up to a maximum of 100mg/day. Wait 1–2 hours after injection to assess response.
6. Amylobarbitone is a powerful respiratory depressant with no pharmacological antagonist. Have facilities for mechanical ventilation available. Amylobarbitone should only be used on the advice of a consultant psychiatrist.
7. Give zuclopenthixol acetate only if repeated IM doses of simple neuroleptics and/or benzodiazepine are required. Onset of action is delayed for 2–8 hours. Effective for 24–36 hours. Do not repeat within 24 hours of previous dose.
   NB. Haloperidol is often appropriate – haloperidol 5–10mg IM acts in 1 or 2 hours and lasts for 18–24 hours.
8. Paraldehyde is now used extremely rarely and is difficult to obtain. It should be used when all else has failed. In many cases, ECT may be more appropriate.

Notes

✧ Recommendations are based partly on clinical experience, partly on theoretical considerations and partly on research data. For review see: Kerr IB, Taylor D. (1997) Acute disturbed or violent behaviour: principles of treatment. *J Psychopharmacol*, **11**, 271–277. Other references include:

Dubin WR. (1988) Rapid tranquillisation: antipsychotics of benzodiazepines. *J Clin Psychiatry*, **49 (suppl. 12)**, 5–11.
Pilowsky LS, Ring H, Shine PJ, *et al.* (1992) Rapid tranquillisation. A survey of emergency prescribing in a general psychiatric hospital. *Br J Psychiatry*, **160**, 831–835.
Resnick M & Burton BT. (1984) Droperidol vs haloperidol in the initial management of acutely agitated patients. *J Clin Psychiatry*, **45**, 298–299.

✧ When available, atypical IM therapy with olanzapine or ziprasidone may be more appropriate than droperidol or haloperidol. No published data as yet but conference posters are encouraging.

See:
Reeves KR, Swift RH. (1998[b]) Rapid-acting, intramuscular ziprasidone 10mg and 20mg in patients with psychosis and acute agitation: results of two double-blind, randomized, fixed-dose studies. *European Psychiatry*, **13**, S304.
Jewell H, Mitchell M, Hatcher B, *et al.* A preliminary study of the safety, efficacy, and pharmacokinetics of intramuscular (IM) olanzapine in patients with acute non-organic psychosis. *Poster presented at International Congress on Schizophrenia Research Biennial Meeting, April 1999, Sante Fe, New Mexico.*

Rapid tranquillisation – monitoring

After any parenteral drug administration monitor as follows:

> **Temperature**
> **Pulse**
> **Blood pressure**
> **Respiratory Rate**
>
> Every 5–10 minutes for one
> hour, then half-hourly until
> patient is ambulatory

If patient is **unconscious**, monitor as above **and** monitor:

> Oxygen saturation
> (by pulse oximetry*)
> continuously until
> ambulatory

*Where available (but strongly recommended).

NB.
ECG monitoring is also strongly recommended when parenteral antipsychotics are given, especially when higher doses are used. Staff should be sufficiently well trained to interpret ECG traces (including calculation of QT/QTc interval).

References

Appleby L, Thomas S, Ferrier N, *et al.* (2000) Sudden unexplained death in psychiatric in-patients. *Br J Psychiatry*, **176**, 405–406.
Yap YG, Camm J. (2000) Risk of torsades de pointes with non-cardiac drugs. *BMJ*, **320**, 1158–1159.

Remedial measures in rapid tranquillisation

Problem	Remedial measures
Acute dystonia (including oculogyric crises)	Give **procyclidine** 5–10mg IM or IV
Reduced respiratory rate (<10/min) or oxygen saturation (<90%)	Give **flumazenil** if benzodiazepine-induced respiratory depression suspected (see protocol) If induced by any other sedative agent: **ventilate mechanically**.
Irregular or slow (<50/min) **pulse**	**Refer** to specialist medical care immediately.
Fall in blood pressure (othostatic or <50mmHg diastolic)	**Lie patient flat**, tilt bed towards head. Monitor closely.
Increased temperature	**Withhold antipsychotics**: (risk of NMS and perhaps arrhythmias)

Guidelines for the use of flumazenil

Indication for use	If, after the administration of lorazepam or diazepam, respiratory rate falls below 10/minute.
Contra-indications	Patients with epilepsy who have been receiving long-term benzodiazepines.
Caution	Dose should be carefully titrated in hepatic impairment.
Dose and route of administration	***Initial:*** 200mcg ***intravenously*** over 15 seconds – if required level of consciousness not achieved after 60 seconds then, ***Subsequent dose:*** 100mcg over 10 seconds.
Time before dose can be repeated	60 seconds.
Maximum dose	1mg in 24 hours (one initial dose and eight subsequent doses).
Side effects	Patients may become agitated, anxious or fearful on awakening.
Management	Side effects usually subside.
Monitoring ❖ **What to monitor?** ❖ **How often?**	 Respiratory rate Continuously until respiratory rate returns to baseline level. *NB. If respiratory rate does not return to normal or patient is not alert after initial doses given then assume sedation due to some other cause.*

Guidelines for the use of Clopixol Acuphase (zuclopenthixol acetate)

When should Clopixol Acuphase be used?

❖ Only after an acutely psychotic patient has required repeated injections of short-acting antipsychotic drugs such as droperidol, or sedative drugs such as lorazepam.

❖ Acuphase should only be given when enough time has elapsed to assess the response to previously injected drugs : allow 15–30 minutes after IV injections; 30–60 minutes after IM.

When should Clopixol Acuphase <u>not</u> be used?

Acuphase should <u>never</u> be administered:

❖ In an attempt to 'hasten' the antipsychotic effect of other antipsychotic therapy

❖ For rapid tranquillisation

❖ At the same time as other parenteral antipsychotics or benzodiazepines

❖ At the same as depot medication

❖ As a 'test dose' for zuclopenthixol decanoate depot

Acuphase should <u>never</u> be used for, or in, the following:

❖ Patients who accept oral medication

❖ Patients who are neuroleptic–naïve

❖ Patients who are sensitive to EPSE

❖ Patients who resist injection (i.e are struggling)

❖ Patients who are in a comatose state

❖ Patients who are pregnant

❖ Those with hepatitis or renal impairment

❖ Those with cardiac disease

How soon does Acuphase take effect?
Sedative effects usually begin to be seen 2 hours after injection and peak after 12 hours. The effects may last for up to 72 hours.

What is the dose?
Acuphase should be given in a dose of 50–150mg, up to a maximum of 400mg in two weeks.

NB Injections should be spaced at least 24 hours apart

VII

Adverse Effects of

Psychotropic Drugs

Guidelines for the management of weight change in patients on psychotropic medication

General considerations:

+ Weight change is a common problem in patients on psychotropic medication with weight gain occurring in approximately 60% of patients on lithium, and 25-50% of patients on valproate, antipsychotics and antidepressants.

+ Weight gain generally occurs because calorie intake exceeds calorie expenditure. This may occur because of actions on a variety of receptors, which can affect hunger and thirst mechanisms, carbohydrate and lipid storage and other metabolic factors. Adverse effects of the drugs may also play a role e.g. lithium-induced hypothyroidism, sedation caused by some antipsychotics. In most instances of weight change with psychotropics, the mechanism remains to be elucidated.

+ Weight gain and weight loss have potentially serious health ramifications in addition to the cosmetic distress often expressed by the patient and is also a frequent cause of poor compliance of medications. The patient's concerns about weight change with respect to their medication should be asked about routinely in all patients on psychotropic medication. Patients are often unwell at the start of treatment, so this discussion should continue as they recover. Motivation and degree of concern about weight are key factors in determining compliance and should be discussed.

+ When considering a subjective complaint of weight change, it is important to consider the natural history of the illness itself, the temporal relationship of the weight problem as well as the relative weight change with respect to height and to original and ideal or 'healthy' body weight.

+ It is important to consider other possible causes in the management of suspected weight change in patients on psychotropics. TSH should be measured, as thyroid abnormalities may be associated with various mental state changes and as some drugs may cause thyroid dysfunction (e.g. carbamazepine, lithium). Some other aetiologies for weight change which should be considered include the following:

weight loss: anorexia nervosa, hypophagia due to depression, delusions concerning food in psychosis, obsessions or ruminations about food in anxiety disorders, underlying neoplasia or other serious medical illness, thyroid dysfunction, unusually restrictive diets.

weight gain: hyperphagia occurring in depression or related to psychosocial stresses, weight gain occurring as a normal part of recovery in depression, thyroid dysfunction, recent smoking discontinuation, oedema or ascites from medical illness (primary or secondary to effects of medications), polydipsia (related to medical or psychiatric illness or to the effects of medication), pregnancy (occurring independently of medication or secondary to oral contraceptive failure due to enzyme-inducing agents e.g. carbamazepine).

+ Consider risk factors, where known. Lithium and valproate have weight gain associated with a predisposition to gain weight, female sex and dose and duration of therapy. Risk factors for antidepressants and antipsychotics have not been yet elucidated.

◆ Consider the individual risk of a given drug for weight change (see table).

◆ All weight changes thought secondary to psychotropics should be discussed fully with the patient. Discussion should continue through recovery, as they may be unwell at the start of therapy. Weight gain from psychotropics often plateaus after a few months and it may thus not always be helpful to switch to an alternative psychotropic. If it is decided to switch to an alternative treatment because of weight change, the patient must be informed of the risk of illness relapse and of other side effects with alternative medications before hand.

◆ Stimulants and other anorexants are not recommended as treatment for side effects of weight gain with psychotropics. Surgical strategies are also not generally recommended as a solution. The use of fluoxetine or of orlistat (tetrahydrolipstatin) may be possible interventions, but neither has been evaluated in this clinical situation.

◆ The use of steroids or body building preparations are not recommended in the treatment of weight loss as a side effect of psychotropics. Such preparations may exacerbate psychiatric symptoms in addition to their other well-known side effects. Patients should be referred wherever possible to a dietician for management of weight loss.

◆ Patients should be referred to a dietician for weight change related to psychotropics, mental status allowing. The patient must also be motivated for such a referral. Fad diets should be avoided. Low fat, high fibre diets maximising fruits and vegetables and complex (over simple) carbohydrates are recommended. Frequency of eating should be considered and thirst as a side effect should be identified, addressing consumption of sugary drinks specifically. This may be a particular risk factor for weight gain with lithium, but may also occur with other medications. As concordance with diets is often difficult, this is best done in conjunction with a behavioural programme and with biofeedback where appropriate.

◆ Exercise is also essential for the management of weight gain: 10-15 minutes/day of exercise may assist the weight loss regime and is best worked into the patient's usual activities of daily living. Note that increased use of calorific energy is possible without 'exercise'. Simply increasing physical activity is effective (e.g. walking instead of catching a bus). Many people are fearful of 'exercise' but will readily increase level of activity in daily living. The aim is to burn off calories, not to build olympic athletes.

Psychotropics and weight change

Drug class	Drugs causing weight gain	Drugs causing weight loss	Drugs thought not to influence weight
Antidepressants	Amitriptyline Imipramine, other TCAs Isocarboxazid Phenelzine ?Tranylcypromine	Fluoxetine ? Bupropion	SSRIs, Moclobemide Venlafaxine Trazodone Nefazodone Amoxapine
Antipsychotics	Phenothiazines Depot preparations Haloperidol Clozapine Olanzapine Quetiapine Risperidone Zotepine	None	Molindone (not available in UK) Loxapine ?Perphenazine Ziprasidone (not licensed in UK at time of publication)
Anxiolytics	None	None	Benzodiazepines
Mood stabilisers / antiepileptic drugs	Lithium Sodium Valproate Vigabatrin ?Carbamazepine	Topiramate, Felbamate	Lamotrigine Gabapentin Phenobarbitone Phenytoin
Stimulants	None	Amphetamines Methylphenidate	? Modafinil

✦ *Antidepressants:* The previous reports of body weight increase by antidepressants were probably overestimates of the problem as weight gain may be a normal part of recovery from depression in some individuals. While one third to one half of patients on tricyclics may experience weight gain, this is usually only modest. Amitriptyline appears to carry the highest risk of TCAs. The non-selective MAOIs also carry significant risk of weight gain and these effects may be additive if used in conjunction with a tricyclic. If weight gain persists, an SSRI or reversible inhibitor of MAO-A (moclobemide) should be considered. Care must be taken to follow the guidelines for switching between these agents. Weight loss appearing during the course of depression is more likely to be related to hypophagia associated with the illness than to be drug-related.

✦ *Mood stabilisers / Antiepileptic Drugs:* Weight gain associated with valproate and lithium as mood stabilisers is common and frequently affects patient concordance with these agents. Although serum lithium levels over 0.8mmol/L are associated with weight gain, lowering of lithium below these levels as a means of weight management cannot be recommended routinely as they will be clinically suboptimal in most patients. Those with identified risk factors should be considered as candidates for carbamazepine, which is less likely to induce weight gain. Thyroid function tests should be checked on any patient on lithium or carbamazepine experiencing weight gain. Lamotrigine and gabapentin are not associated with significant weight gain, but there are too few data concerning their efficacy as mood stabilisers to recommend switching to these agents routinely. The data concerning other AEDs as mood stabilisers are even less convincing.

◆ *Antipsychotics:* Phenothiazines and the newer atypical agents appear to have the greatest risk of weight gain associated with their use. Some have suggested that there is a correlation between treatment efficacy and bodyweight gain for many antipsychotics. There is a theoretical problem with the common use of valproate with clozapine as both may cause significant weight gain, although no clinical studies have addressed this potential problem to date. Of the typical antipsychotics, butyrophenones are less likely than phenothiazines to cause body weight gain and loxapine, molindone and perphenazine do not appear to cause weight gain, although data are scarce. See following section for more specific information.

◆ *Anxiolytics:* Consistent weight changes with anxiolytics have not been demonstrated, and other causes should be sought when weight change occurs in this clinical situation (e.g. co-morbidty with an eating disorder or depression; e.g. thyroid disorder causing anxiety symptoms).

◆ *Stimulants:* Amphetamines and methylphenidate frequently cause weight loss; modafanil has been reported to cause anorexia more commonly than placebo, but there are few data relevant to weight changes with this agent.

References

Ackerman S, Nolan LJ. (1998) Bodyweight gain induced by psychotropic agents: incidence, mechanisms and management. *CNS Drugs,* **9**, 135–151

Isojärvi JIT, Laatikainen TJ, Knip M, *et al.* (1996) Obesity and endocrine disorders in women taking valproate for epilepsy. *Ann Neurol,* **39**, 579–584.

Pijl H, Meinders AE, (1998) Bodyweight Change as an Adverse Effect of Drug Treatment. *Drug Saf,* **14**, 329–342.

Silverstone T. (1996) Body weight changes during treatment with psychotropic drugs (Psychiatrists Information Service Monograph Series No. 1). Janssen Pharmaceuticals, Oxford, UK.

Specific recommendations:

On initial prescription of psychotropics likely to cause weight change:

1. Consider risk factors

2. Discuss pros and cons with patient

3. Monitor weight monthly x 6 months then every 3 months

4. Consider early referral to a dietician, if patient agreeable and mental state appropriate

5. Consider the possible additive effects of weight change effects if this psychotropic is being added to another producing similar weight change

6. Obtain baseline BMI and relevant laboratory parameters (e.g. TFTs)

7. Consider the patient's ideal body weight, any other risk factors for obesity-related illness and the attitude of the patient towards weight gain or loss

---

If weight change does occur, rule out other possible causes:

1. Take careful history, including dietary and family history as well as temporal relationship of weight change to initiation and dose changes of psychotropics

2. Consider the role of thirst which should not be underestimated – in particular all drinks with high sugar content should be excluded

3. Physical examination to include height, weight, calculation of body mass index; look for evidence of ascites, myxoedema

4. Check thyroid function tests, FBC, LFTs, albumin, electrolytes

5. Consider other relevant tests, e.g. pregnancy testing

If other causes of weight change excluded, institute dietary and exercise regime in conjunction with dietician and/or exercise physiologist. Exercise may be undertaken in groups as the psychological benefits of such encouragement are important. The types of exercise chosen must take into account any effects of the medication on alertness or coordination. Increased activity is the ultimate goal.

If above not successful, consider alternative drugs in same class which might have less risk for weight change (see table). However, weight gain often plateaus and so switching may not always be necessary or desirable. Any such change that does occur must take into account the risk of relapse on changing of medication and be fully discussed with the patient with respect to risks and benefits.

Weight gain with antipsychotics

All antipsychotics are liable to cause weight gain

Risk of weight gain	Drug
Very high	Clozapine
High	Olanzapine Thioridazine Zotepine
Medium	Chlorpromazine Risperidone Thioxanthines Quetiapine
Low	Amisulpride/sulpiride Butyrophenones Pimozide Piperazine phenothiazines
Very low	Ziprasidone

Information in this table was derived from a meta-analysis and a systematic review. See:

Allison DB, Mentore JL, Heo M, *et al.* (1999) Antipsychotic-induced weight gain: a comprehensive research synthesis. *Am J Psychiatry,* **156,** 1686–1696.

Taylor D, McAskill R. (2000) Weight gain with atypical antipsychotics – a systematic review. *Acta Psychiatr Scand* **101**, 416–432.

Weight gain with antipsychotics

Advice for prescribers

✦   All antipsychotics can cause weight gain, although risk varies from drug to drug.

✦   Suggested mechanisms include D_2 antagonism, H_1 antagonism and $5HT_{2C}$ antagonism.

✦   Weight gain seems to be caused by increased appetite and food intake.

✦   Time course of weight gain is poorly researched, but most weight gain seems to be in the first 6–9 months of treatment.

✦   Switching to a drug less likely to cause weight gain may, under certain circumstances, be prudent, but research is lacking.

✦   All patients should be advised to take more exercise (walking is ideal), aiming for 20–30 minutes each day.

✦   Where increased appetite is evident or expected, patients should be encouraged to eat fruit and vegetables.

✦   Refer early to a dietician where available.

Weight gain with antipsychotics

Advice for patients and carers

✦ All antipsychotics can cause weight gain, but some drugs are worse than others.

✦ People put on weight because they feel more hungry and eat more.

✦ On average, people taking antipsychotics put on 2–10lb, depending on the drug taken.

✦ Weight gain can probably be avoided by

  ✧ Eating fruit or vegetables instead of confectionery or fast-food.
  ✧ Being more active – walking is ideal, but swimming and team sports are also good. Aim for 20–30 minutes every day.

✦ Switching drugs may help in some cases, but there is no research to prove it.

Antidepressants – relative adverse effects

Drug	Sedation	Cardio-toxicity	Anti-cholinergic effects	Forms available
Tricyclics				
Imipramine	++	+++	+++	tabs, liq
Amitriptyline	+++	+++	+++	tabs/caps, liq, inj
Desipramine*	+	++	+	tabs
Nortriptyline	+	++	+	tabs
Trimipramine	+++	+++	++	tabs, caps
Doxepin	+++	++	++	caps
Dothiepin	+++	+++	++	tabs, caps
Clomipramine	++	+++	++	tabs/caps, liq, inj
Lofepramine	+	+	+	tabs
Atypical antidepressants				
Mirtazapine	+++	- ?	+	tabs
Nefazodone	++	-	-	tabs
Reboxetine	+	- ?	+	tabs
Trazodone	+++	+	-	caps, liq
Venlafaxine	++	- ?	+	tabs
Selective Serotonin Reuptake Inhibitors (SSRIs)				
Citalopram	-	- ?	-	tabs
Fluvoxamine	+	- ?	-	tabs
Fluoxetine	-	-	-	caps, liq
Sertraline	-	-	-	tabs
Paroxetine	+	-	+	tabs, liq
Monoamine Oxidase Inhibitors (MAOIs)				
Isocarboxazid	+	++	++	tabs
Phenelzine	+	+	+	tabs
Tranylcypromine	-	+	+	tabs
Reversible Inhibitor Of Monoamine Oxidase A (RIMA)				
Moclobemide	-	-	-	tabs

KEY:
+++ High incidence/severity
++ Moderate
* In UK, available on named-patient basis only

- Very low/none
+ Low

Antipsychotics – relative adverse effects

Drug	Sedation	Extra-pyramidal	Anti-cholinergic	Hypotension	Cardiac toxicity	Prolactin elevation
Chlorpromazine	+++	++	++	+++	++	+++
Promazine	+++	+	++	++	+	++
Thioridazine	+++	+	+++	+++	+++	++
Fluphenazine	+	+++	++	+	+	+++
Perphenazine	+	+++	+	+	+	+++
Trifluoperazine	+	+++	+/ -	+	+	+++
Flupenthixol	+	++	++	+	+	+++
Zuclopenthixol	++	++	++	+	+	+++
Haloperidol	+	+++	+	+	+	+++
Droperidol	++	+++	+	+	+	+++
Benperidol	+	+++	+	+	+	+++
Sulpiride	-	+	+/ -	-	-	+++
Pimozide	+	+	+	+	+++	+++
Loxapine	++	+++	+	++	+	+++
Clozapine	+++	-	+++	+++	+	-
Risperidone	+	+	+	++	-	+++
Sertindole*	-	-	-	+++	+++	-
Olanzapine	++	+/ -	+	+	-	+
Quetiapine	++	-	+	++	-	-
Amisulpride	-	+	-	-	-	+++
Zotepine	+++	++	+	++	++	++
Ziprasidone**	+	+/ -	-	+	+	+

Key: +++ High incidence/ severity   ++ Moderate
          + Low   - Very low
* Named patient only
** Not licensed in UK at time of publication

Clozapine – management of adverse effects

Adverse effect	Timecourse	Action
Sedation	First 4 weeks. May persist, but usually wears off	Give smaller dose in the mornings. Some patients can only cope with single night-time dosing. Reduce dose if necessary
Hypersalivation	First 4 weeks. May persist, but usually wears off. Often very troublesome at night	Give hyoscine 300mcg (Kwells) sucked and swallowed at night. Pirenzepine (not licensed in the UK) up to 50mg tds may be tried. Patients do not always mind excess salivation: treatment not always required
Constipation	Usually persists	Recommend high fibre diet. Bulk forming laxatives +/-stimulants may be used
Hypotension	First 4 weeks	Advise patient to take time when standing up. Reduce dose or slow down rate of increase. If severe, consider moclobemide and Bovril, or fludrocortisone
Hypertension	First 4 weeks, sometimes longer	Monitor closely and increase dose as slowly as is necessary. Hypotensive therapy (e.g. atenolol 25mg/day) is rarely necessary
Tachycardia	First 4 weeks, but often persists	Often occurs if dose escalation is too rapid. Inform patient that it is not dangerous. Give small dose of beta-blocker if necessary
Weight gain	Usually during the first year of treatment	Dietary counselling is essential. Advice may be more effective if given before weight gain occurs. Weight gain is common and often profound (10lb +)
Fever	First 3 weeks	Give antipyretic but check FBC. NB. This fever is not usually related to blood dyscrasias
Seizures	May occur at any time	Dose /dose increase related. Consider prophylactic valproate* if on high dose. After a seizure – withhold clozapine for one day. Restart at reduced dose. Give sodium valproate
Nausea	First 6 weeks	May give anti-emetic. Avoid prochlorperazine and metoclopramide if previous EPSE
Nocturnal enuresis	May occur at any time	Try manipulating dose schedule. Avoid fluids before bedtime. In severe cases, desmopressin is usually effective
Neutropenia/ agranulocytosis	First 18 weeks (but may occur at any time)	Stop clozapine; admit to hospital

* Usual dose is 1000-2000mg/day. Plasma levels may be useful as a rough guide to dosing – aim for 50-100mg/L. Use of modified release preparation (Epilim Chrono) may aid compliance: can be given once daily and may be better tolerated.

References

Fritze J, Tilmann E. (1995) Pirenzepine for clozapine-induced hypersalivation. *Lancet*, **346**, 1034.

Pacia SV, Devinsky O. (1994) Clozapine-related seizures: experience with 5,629 patients. *Neurology*, **44**, 2247–2249.

Taylor D, Reveley A, Faivre F. (1995) Clozapine-induced hypotension treated with moclobemide and Bovril. *Br J Psychiatry*, **167**, 409–410.

Clozapine – serious adverse effects

Agranulocytosis, thromboembolism, cardiomyopathy and myocarditis

Clozapine very clearly and substantially *reduces* overall mortality in schizophrenia, largely because of a considerable reduction in the rate of suicide.[1,2]

Nevertheless, clozapine can cause serious, life-threatening adverse effects of which **agranulocytosis** is the best known. In the UK, there have been three deaths due to clozapine-associated agranulocytosis – a risk of 1 in 4,250 patients treated. Risk is well managed by the CPMS.

A possible association between clozapine and **pulmonary embolism** has recently been emphasised. Initially, Walker and co-workers[1] uncovered a risk of fatal pulmonary embolism of 1 in 4,500 – about 20 times the risk in the population as a whole. Following a case report of non-fatal pulmonary embolism possibly related to clozapine,[3] data from the Swedish authorities were recently presented.[4] Twelve cases of venous thromboembolism were described, of which five were fatal. The risk of thromboembolism was estimated to be 1 in 2,000–6,000 patients treated. Thromboembolism may be related to clozapine's observed effect on antiphospholipid antibodies.[5] It seems most likely to occur in the first three months of treatment.

It has also been suggested that clozapine is associated with **myocarditis** and **cardiomyopathy**. Most recently, Australian data identified 23 cases (15 myocarditis, 8 cardiomyopathy) of which 6 were fatal.[6] Risk of death from either cause is estimated from these data to be 1 in 1,300. Myocarditis seems to occur within three weeks of starting clozapine.

It is notable that other data sources give rather different risk estimates: in Canada the risk of fatal myocarditis was estimated to be 1 in 12,500, and in the USA, 1 in 67,000.[7]

Note also that, despite an overall reduction in mortality, younger patients may have an increased risk of sudden death[8] perhaps because of clozapine-induced ECG changes.[9] The overall picture remains very unclear but caution is required. There may, of course, be similar problems with other antipsychotics.[10]

Summary

❖ Mortality in schizophrenia is around 100% higher than the general population.

❖ Mortality in those treated with clozapine is about 75% higher than the general population.

❖ Risk of fatal agranulocytosis is around 1 in 4,250 patients treated under the Clozaril Patient Monitoring Scheme.

❖ Risk of fatal pulmonary embolism is estimated to be around 1 in 4,500 patients treated.

❖ Risk of fatal myocarditis or cardiomyopathy may be as high as 1 in 1,300 patients treated.

❖ Careful monitoring is essential especially during the first three months of treatment.

References

1. Walker AM. (1997) Mortality in current and former users of clozapine. *Epidemiology*, **8**, 671–677.
2. Munro J, O'Sullivan D, Andrews C, *et al.* (1999) Active monitoring of 12,760 clozapine recipients in the UK and Ireland: Beyond pharmacovigilance. *Br J Psychiatry*, **175**, 576–580.
3. Lacika S, Cooper JP. (1999) Pulmonary embolus possibly associated with clozapine treatment. *Can J Psychiatry*, **44**, 396–397 (Letter).
4. Hägg S, Spigset O, Söderström TG. (2000) Association of venous thromboembolism and clozapine. *Lancet*, **355**, 1155–1156.
5. Davis S. (1994) Antiphospholipid antibodies associated with clozapine treatment. *Am J Hematol*, **46**, 166–167.
6. Kilian JG, Kerr K, Lawrence C, *et al.* (1999) Myocarditis and cardiomyopathy associated with clozapine. *Lancet*, **354**, 1841–1845.
7. Warner B, Alphs L, Schaedelin J, *et al.* (2000) Myocarditis and cardiomyopathy associated with clozapine. *Lancet*, **355**, 842–843 (Letter).
8. Modal I, Hirschman S, Rava A, *et al.* (2000) Sudden death in patients receiving clozapine treatment: a preliminary investigation. *J Clin Psychopharmacol*, **20**, 325–327.
9. Kang UG, Kwon JS, Ahn YM, *et al.* (2000) Electrocardiographic abnormalities in patients treated with clozapine. *J Clin Psychiatry*, **61**, 441–446.
10. Thomassen R, Vandenbroucke JP, Rosendaal FR. (2000) Antipsychotic drugs and thromboembolism. *Lancet*, **356**, 252 (letter).

Algorithm for the treatment of antipsychotic-induced akathisia

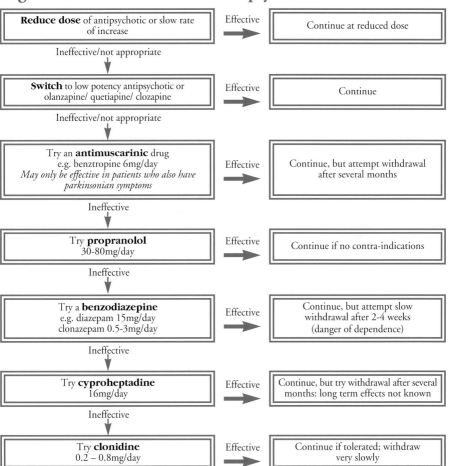

Reduce dose of antipsychotic or slow rate of increase	Effective →	Continue at reduced dose

Ineffective/not appropriate ↓

Switch to low potency antipsychotic or olanzapine/ quetiapine/ clozapine	Effective →	Continue

Ineffective/not appropriate ↓

Try an **antimuscarinic** drug e.g. benztropine 6mg/day *May only be effective in patients who also have parkinsonian symptoms*	Effective →	Continue, but attempt withdrawal after several months

Ineffective ↓

Try **propranolol** 30-80mg/day	Effective →	Continue if no contra-indications

Ineffective ↓

Try a **benzodiazepine** e.g. diazepam 15mg/day clonazepam 0.5-3mg/day	Effective →	Continue, but attempt slow withdrawal after 2-4 weeks (danger of dependence)

Ineffective ↓

Try **cyproheptadine** 16mg/day	Effective →	Continue, but try withdrawal after several months: long term effects not known

Ineffective ↓

Try **clonidine** 0.2 – 0.8mg/day	Effective →	Continue if tolerated; withdraw very slowly

Notes

⬦ Akathisia is sometimes difficult to diagnose with certainty. A careful history of symptoms and drug use is essential. Note that severe akathisia may be linked to violent behaviour.

⬦ Evaluate efficacy of each treatment option over at least one month. Some effect may be seen after a few days but it may take much longer to become apparent in those with chronic akathisia.

⬦ Withdraw previously ineffective treatments before starting the next option in the algorithm.

⬦ Consider tardive akathisia in patients on long term therapy.

References

Adler L, Angrist B, Peselow E, *et al.* (1986) A controlled assessment of propranolol in the treatment of neuroleptic-induced akathisia. *Br J Psychiatry*, **149**, 42–45.

Fleischhacker WW, Roth SD, Kane JM. (1990) The pharmacologic treatment of neuroleptic-induced akathisia. *J Clin Psychopharmacol*, **10**, 12–21.

Weiss D, Aizenberg D, Hermesh H, *et al.* (1995) Cyproheptadine treatment of neuroleptic-induced akathisia. *Br J Psychiatry*, **167**, 483–486.

Algorithm for the treatment of symptomatic, antipsychotic-induced hyperprolactinaemia

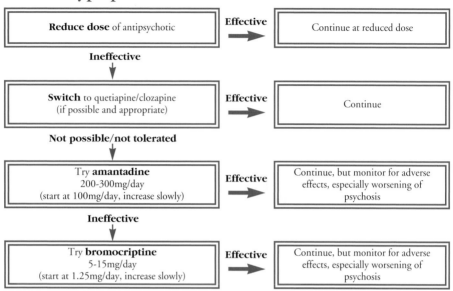

Notes

◇ Hyperprolactinaemia is often asymptomatic. Adverse effects, when they do occur, are sometimes mild and do not affect quality of life. Remedial treatment is therefore only occasionally appropriate. In cases of apparent infertility, specialist advice should be sought.

◇ Before starting treatment – take a full sexual/menstrual history to establish whether or not symptoms are related to antipsychotic use.

◇ Other causes of hyperprolactinaemia (eg prolactin-secreting tumour) must be considered.

◇ Evaluate efficacy of each treatment option over at least one month: prolactin levels may fall within days but adverse effects such as gynaecomastia respond more slowly.

◇ Withdraw previously ineffective treatments before starting the next option in the algorithm.

◇ Olanzapine causes dose-dependent, transient hyperprolactinaemia. Symptoms are rare, especially at 10mg/day. Ziprasidone, too, has minimal effects on prolactin.

Modified from Duncan and Taylor (1995). Treatment of psychotropic-induced hyperprolactinaemia, *Psych Bull*, **19**, 755–757.

The neuroleptic malignant syndrome (NMS)

- Incidence: 0.5 – 1% patients

- Mortality (untreated) 20%

- Onset may be acute or insidious

- Course may fluctuate

- May occur out of hospital

SIGNS AND SYMPTOMS

⬦ Intense diaphoresis
⬦ Fever/hyperthermia
⬦ Hypertension/autonomic instability (fluctuating B.P.)
⬦ Tachycardia
⬦ Incontinence / retention / obstruction
⬦ Muscular rigidity (may be confined to head and neck)
⬦ Confusion, agitation/altered consciousness
⬦ Raised creatinine phosphokinase > 1000 IU/L (controversial)
⬦ Leukocytosis

RISK FACTORS

⬦ Organic brain disease: alcoholism, dementia
⬦ Hypermetabolic states: hyperthyroidism
⬦ Psychiatric diagnosis
⬦ Parkinsons' disease
⬦ Agitation
⬦ Dehydration
⬦ History of catatonia
⬦ High dose antipsychotic
⬦ Recent dose increase

PRECIPITATING FACTORS

⬦ Antipsychotics: typical and atypical
⬦ Rapidity of titration and dose of drug
⬦ Antipsychotic withdrawal
⬦ Antidepressants: including SSRIs
⬦ Abrupt cessation of dopamine agonists
⬦ Other drugs: tetrabenazine
⬦ Drugs of abuse: cocaine, MDMA, amphetamine

TREATMENTS

✧ Withdraw antipsychotic immediately
✧ General supportive medical intervention on medical ward
✧ Rehydration
✧ Sedation with short-acting benzodiazepines
✧ Dopamine agonists: bromocriptine, dantrolene
✧ Antimuscarinic agents
✧ Propranolol
✧ Electroconvulsive therapy
✧ Plasmaphoresis

COMPLICATIONS

✧ Renal: rhabdomyolysis leading to renal failure
✧ Cardiovascular: arrythmias, cardiac arrest, stroke, cardiogenic shock
✧ Respiratory: respiratory failure, pulmonary embolus
✧ Hepatic failure
✧ E.coli fasciitis

Antipsychotic rechallenge

✦ Antipsychotic rechallenge following NMS is associated with an acceptable risk in most patients

✦ Gender and age do not affect successful rechallenge

✦ A minimum of 5–14 days should elapse post recovery

✦ Generally, successful rechallenge uses structurally dissimilar agents

✦ Lower doses are recommended, with extremely slow titration

✦ Depot preparations should be avoided

✦ Agents with lower D_2 receptor blockade may be preferred, but data are inconclusive

References

Koponen H, Repo E, Lepola U. (1991) Long-term outcome after neuroleptic malignant syndrome. *Acta Psychiatr Scand*, **84**, 550–551.
Levenson JL. (1985) Neuroleptic malignant syndrome. *Am J Psychiatry*, **142**, 1137–1145.
Lishman WA. (1998) Organic Psychiatry, Third Edition. Blackwell Science, London, U.K.
Modestin J, Toffler G, Drescher JP. (1992) Neuroleptic malignant syndrome: results of a prospective study. *Psychiatry Res*, **44**, 251–256.
Spivak B, Gonen N, Mester R, *et al*. (1996) Neuroleptic malignant syndrome associated with abrupt withdrawal of anticholinergic agents. *Int Clin Psychopharmacol*, **11**, 207–209.
Wells AJ, Sommi RW, Crismon ML. (1988) Neuroleptic rechallenge after neuroleptic malignant syndrome case report and literature review. *Drug Intell Clin Pharm*, **22**, 475–480.

Algorithm for the treatment of tardive dyskinesia (TD)

Prevention whenever possible	✧ consider risk factors e.g. females, the elderly, affective disorder, total antipsychotic dose — use lowest dose of antipsychotic for shortest time necessary — reassess need for antipsychotic regularly e.g. three monthly — reassess need for antimuscarinic regularly — consider use of antipsychotic less likely to cause TD
If TD develops withdraw any antimuscarinic **Consider withdrawing antipsychotic slowly**	✧ antimuscarinic withdrawal may allow improvement in TD ✧ balance risk of relapse against risk of TD ✧ TD is not usually progressive ✧ continuing at the lowest possible dose minimises the risk of progression

Antipsychotic required

If antipsychotic necessary consider clozapine (or olanzapine or quetiapine)	✧ clozapine may allow improvement in TD ✧ consider using mood stabilisers alone for bipolar disorder

Further measures

Consider Vitamin E 400iu/day; may increase by 400iu weekly to a maximum of 1600iu/day in divided doses	✧ consider withdrawing other drugs which may cause or exacerbate movement disorders e.g. metoclopramide, antidepressants, stimulants, antimuscarinics and antiparkinsonian agents ✧ monitor for GI effects of Vitamin E ✧ treatment duration is not clearly established ✧ some doubt over efficacy

TD persists

Consider clonazepam 1mg/day (elderly 0.5mg) and ↑ over 2-4 weeks to 4.5mg/day	✧ tolerance to clonazepam may develop; therefore intermittent treatment is preferable ✧ dystonia may respond better

TD persists

✧ Other proposed treatments Consider: ✧ Nifedipine 40 – 80mg[1]/day ✧ Sodium Valproate[2] ✧ Ondansetron 12mg/day ✧ Propanolol – for tardive akathisia ✧ Botulinum toxin – for tardive dystonia ✧ Tetrabenazine – A/E limit use e.g. depression ✧ Increasing antipsychotic dose[3]	1. maybe more effective in elderly and in severe TD 2. some evidence of efficacy ?prophylactic use 3. will improve TD initially but will worsen TD in long term

N.B. Symptoms of TD occur in untreated schizophrenia: antipsychotics are not the only risk factor.

References

Adler LA, Rotrosen J, Edson R, *et al.* (1999) Vitamin E treatment for tardive dyskinesia. *Arch Gen Psychiatry*, **56**, 836–841.

Beasley CM, Dellva MA, Tamura RN. (1999) Randomised double-blind comparison of the incidence of tardive dyskinesia in patients with schizophrenia during long-term treatment with olanzapine or haloperidol. *Br J Psychiatry*, **174**, 23–30.

Caligiuri MP, Lacro JP, Rockwell E, *et al.* (1997) Incidence and risk factors for severe tardive dyskinesia in older patients. *Br J Psychiatry*, **171**, 148–153.

Cavallaro, R, Smeraldi E. (1995) Antipsychotic-induced tardive dyskinesia. *CNS Drugs*, **4**, 278–293.

Chakos MH, Alvir JMJ, Woerner MG, *et al.* (1996) Incidence and correlates of tardive dyskinesia in first episode of schizophrenia. *Arch Gen Psychiatry*, **53**, 313–319.

Duncan D, McConnell H, Taylor D. (1977) Tardive dyskinesia – how is it prevented and treated? *Psych Bull*, **21**, 422–425.

Glazer WM. (2000) Expected incidence of tardive dyskinesia associated with atypical antipsychotics. *J Clin Psychiatry*, **61(suppl 4)**, 21–26.

Joseph AB, Young RR. (1992) Movement disorders in neurology and neuropsychiatry and neuropsychiatry. *Scientific Publications,* Oxford.

Keghavan MS, Kennedy JS. (1992) *Drug induced dysfunction in psychiatry.* Hemisphere Publishing, New York.

Kinon BJ, Milton DR, Stauffer VL, *et al.* Effect of chronic olanzapine treatment on the course of presumptive tardive dyskinesia. Presented at American Psychiatric Association 152nd Annual Meeting, May 1999, Washington DC.

Morgenstern H, Glazer WM. (1993) Identifying risk factors for tardive dyskinesia among long-term outpatients maintained with neuroleptic medications. *Arch Gen Psychiatry*, **50**, 723–733.

Simpson GM. (2000) The treatment of tardive dyskinesia and tardive dystonia. *J Clin Psychiatry*, **61(suppl 4)**, 39–44.

Sirota P, Mosheva T, Shabtay H, *et al.* (2000) Use of the selective serotonin 3 receptor antagonist ondansetron in the treatment of neuroleptic-induced tardive dyskinesia. *Am J Psychiatry*, **157**, 287–289.

Soutullo CA, Keck PE, McElroy SL. (1999) Olanzapine in the treatment of tardive dyskinesia: a report of two cases. *J Clin Psychopharmacol*, **19**, 100–101 (Letter).

Toenniessen LM, Casey DE, McFarland BH. (1985) Tardive dyskinesia in the aged: duration of treatment relationships. *Arch Gen Psychiatry*, **42**, 278–284.

Van Os J, Fahy T, Jones P, *et al.* (1997) Tardive dyskinesia: who is at risk? *Acta Psychiatr Scan*, **96**, 206–216.

Vesely C, Küfferle B, Brücke T, *et al.* (2000) Remission of severe tardive dyskinesia in a schizophrenic patient treated with the atypical antipsychotic substance quetiapine. *Int Clin Psychopharmacol*, **15**, 57–60.

Appendices

Appendix I

Antibiotic use in psychiatry

General guidelines

❖ Suitable samples of infected material should be sent for microbiological examination before initiating empirical antimicrobial therapy. Contact Microbiology for advice about sampling and therapy.

❖ BNF doses should be followed.

❖ When appropriate, oral therapy should be instituted. Prescriptions should be for a 5 day course and then reviewed. However, in the case of chronic diseases which require long term therapy, e.g. osteomyelitis, neurosyphilis or tuberculosis, advice should be sought from the Infection Control Team or other appropriate specialists.

❖ If after 48 hours' therapy clinical improvement is not observed, or treatment shown to be inappropriate, Microbiology should be consulted.

❖ [i] Intravenous/intramuscular antibiotics are not listed and will usually not be reported as many Psychiatric nursing staff are not qualified to administer them. However where these routes are considered essential, please contact Microbiology, Pharmacy, or other appropriate specialists.

[ii] The circumstances in which the parenteral route should be considered are if:

a] the patient is seriously ill,

b] the infection is sensitive to a parenteral-only agent,

c] the infection has not responded to an appropriate course of oral therapy,

d] the patient is unable to take medication orally.

❖ Topical antibiotics, including mupirocin should be avoided unless recommended by the Infection Control Team or other appropriate specialists.

❖ Where the oral route is contraindicated, metronidazole can be administered rectally. Please contact Microbiology or Pharmacy.

❖ Infected samples of urine from patients who are catheterised should not lead to automatic treatment unless systemic infection is present. Consult Microbiology.

❖ Products to which the patients are known to be allergic should NEVER be administered. NB. Allergy to penicillins is rarely associated with cross sensitivity to cephalosporins. If in doubt contact Microbology or Pharmacy.

Recommended treatment of common infections

For urinary tract infections [UTI]:

1st line: trimethoprim, amoxycillin or cefadroxil.
2nd line: nalidixic acid or co-amoxiclav.
Multiple resistant organisms: ciprofloxacin.

For respiratory tract infections:

1st line: amoxycillin or erythromycin. If not improving in 24 hours, consult Microbiology.
2nd line: clarithromycin [3 day course] or co-amoxiclav.

For fungal infections:

Nystatin suspension for oral infections; clotrimazole for skin infections;
fluconazole for systemic or resistant skin infections.
Terbinafine may be used in some instances. Consult Microbiology.

For throat infections - Streps:

Penicillin, erythromycin or amoxycillin.

For wounds / ulcers and pressure sores: topical antibiotics may not be used. In most cases wound irrigation and cleaning are sufficient. If there are clinical signs and symptoms of cellulitis consult Microbiology.

For pelvic inflammatory disease and vaginal discharge:

Collect high vaginal swab. If Neisseria gonorrhoeae [the gonococcus, GC] is excluded, treat:
1st line: metronidazole [400mg bd for 5-7 days] PLUS doxycycline [100mg bd for 14 days].
Erythromycin may be substituted for doxycycline if doxycycline is not tolerated [500mg qds for 14 days].
For GC consult Microbiology.

For gastroenteritis:

Antibiotics are not generally indicated. The Infection Control Team or other appropriate specialist must be informed and faecal samples must be sent to the laboratory.

For eyes and ears - topical:

For advice, particularly if otitis media is suspected, consult Microbiology or Pathology.
Eyes - 1st line: chloramphenicol drops/ointment.
Ears - 1st line: chloramphenicol drops. [2nd line: neomycin, polymyxin].

For tuberculosis

A chest physician must be consulted for recommendations. Tuberculosis is a notifiable disease and the Infection Control Team must be alerted immediately if the disease is suspected.

Treatment of specific organisms

For Staph aureus:

Flucloxacillin, or sodium fusidate PLUS erythromycin.

For MRSA:

Contact the Infection Control Team or other appropriate specialist and see the MRSA policy in the current Infection Control Policy for suitable topical preparations and protocols for treatment of colonisation and infection.

For Anaerobes:

Metronidazole.

First Line Agents

Antibiotic	Form	Strength	Usual dose
AMOXYCILLIN	capsules suspension	250mg 250mg/5ml	250-500mg tds
CEFADROXIL	capsules suspension	500mg 500mg /5ml	500mg bd
DOXYCYCLINE	capsules	100mg	200mg stat, 100mg od
ERYTHROMYCIN	tablets	250mg	250-500mg qds/tds
FLUCLOXACILLIN	capsules	250mg	250-500mg qds
METRONIDAZOLE	tablets suppositories	200mg 1g	200-400mg tds 1g tds x 3/7 then bd
TRIMETHOPRIM	tablets	200mg	200mg bd

Antifungal	Form	Strength	Usual dose
* Nystatin	mouthwash	100,000 units/ml	1ml qds
Fluconazole	capsules	50mg	50mg od
Clotrimazole	pessaries	500mg	one stat.

[* topical effect only: not absorbed systemically]

Second Line Agents

Recommended by Microbiology in the case of resistant organisms

Antibiotic	Form	Strength	Usual dose
CIPROFLOXACIN	tablets	250mg	250mg bd
CO-AMOXICLAV	tablets	375mg	1 tds
NALIDIXIC ACID	tablet	500mg	1g qds
SODIUM FUSIDATE	tablets	250mg	500mg tds
TEICOPLANIN	injection	200mg	400mg stat, 200mg/d

Note

These guidelines were developed specifically for the South London and Maudsley NHS Trust and may be different in many respects from policies in other hospitals. Always consult Microbiology, Pathology or Pharmacy departments if in any doubt about antibiotic prescribing.

Appendix II

Communication with service users

Follow the CAAT system:

Consultative

Those being prescribed medication should be consulted about their preferences with regard to adverse effects and likely outcomes with different medication. Patients' informed preferences should influence drug choice. Ideally, patients themselves should choose which medication they are prescribed. When patients are too ill to be consulted about drug choice, the opportunity for informative discussion should be provided as soon as is appropriate

Accurate

Patients have the right to factually accurate information about medicines and prescribing choices. Healthcare workers should recognise the limits of their knowledge and refer to expert advice when necessary. Consider, also, the provision of written information and patient telephone helplines.

Appropriate

Information should be presented in such a way that it can be readily understood. It is more important to tell patients how medication affects symptoms than to try to explain complex theories of drug action. It is rarely necessary to discuss, for instance, receptor theory, but likely outcomes should certainly be discussed. Everyone should be afforded the opportunity to be given more information, having first reflected on the information initially provided or after having gained first-hand experience of medication prescribed.

True

Patients have the right to be told the truth about medicines. It is morally right to impart all *relevant* information to those prescribed medication. Being 'economical with the truth' is unethical and likely to damage relationships and perhaps lead to litigation. Clearly, it is impossible to tell patients everything that is known about a particular medication, but it is possible to direct patients to more comphrehensive, well-grounded sources of information.

MAUDSLEY DISCUSSION PAPERS

1. **The General Practitioner, the Psychiatrist and the Burden of Mental Health Care** (1997)
   (Prof Goldberg & Prof Gournay)

2. **Disputed Confessions and the Criminal Justice System** (1997)
   (Dr Gudjonsson & Dr Mackeith)

3. **Hard to Swallow: Compulsory Treatment in Eating Disorders** (1997)
   (Dr Treasure & Dr Ramsay)

4. **Child and Adolescent Mental Health Services: Reasoned Advice to Commissioners and Practitioners** (1997)
   (Dr R Goodman)

5. **Has Community Care Failed?** (1998)
   (Prof G Thornicroft & Prof D Goldberg)

6. **Should the English Special Hospitals be Closed?** (1998)
   (Prof J Gunn & Prof A Maden)

7. **Should Psychiatrists Treat Personality Disorders?** (1999)
   (Dr P Moran)

8. **Specialist Services for Minority Ethnic Groups?** (2000)
   (Dr K Bhui, Dr D Bhugra & Dr K McKenzie)

9. **Adoption as a Placement Choice: Arguments and Evidence** (2000)
   (Dr Alan Rushton)

10. **Mental Health Law: Discrimination or Protection?** (2000)
    (Dr George Szmukler & Dr Frank Holloway)

All priced at £4 each.

Available from Mrs Sarah Smith, Room M118, The Division of Psychological Medicine, Institute of Psychiatry, de Crespigny Park, London SE5 8AF
Telephone: 020 7848 0140   Fax: 020 7701 9044   E-mail: <u>sarah.smith@iop.kcl.ac.uk</u>

Please make cheques payable to 'King's College London'

*To find out more about these and other Maudsley Publications,
why not visit our web site at http://www.iop.kcl.ac.uk/Main/Publicat.htm*